General Health Guide

gavin morey

traintobecome

Myo Clinic Publishing

www.myoclinic.co.uk

ISBN 978-0-9564955-0-1

Acknowledgements

I don't know where to start, but I would like to thank my family and friends for all their support throughout the past five years on the making of these books. It has been a long and hard process, but it has been well worth it in the end!

I have had a lot of help from my Mum and Dad, you both mean the world to me. To my brothers, Chris, Rob and Aaron, I would like to thank you for keeping me grounded and helping me with the books and website. Thanks to my friend Simon for being there for the past 12 years with all of my silly ideas and enterprises and to Gav, for training with me and keeping me on track all the way to the end. I would also just like to say thank you to Fred for training with me throughout the 12 weeks and helping me with all of my business concerns. You have helped me more than you realise.

Finally, to my beautiful and devoted fiancee, you gave me so much help and support, especially towards the end in writing these books. Thank you and I love you so much x.

Contents

Introduction

The Train to Become General Health Guide is part of a three book collection dedicated to showing you how to change your body and lifestyle in just 12 weeks. This book focuses not only on your lifestyle and your body, but looks at and explains home health tests, postural analysis and recognising your own skin type. And it provides tried and tested methods of counteracting certain skin and body complaints.

As a personal trainer and sports therapist it is very easy for me to dictate to clients how they should live and exercise without even giving it a second thought. But I decided to discover how the average person can indeed become a fitter and healthier version of themselves in a matter of weeks by undergoing a five month period of living unhealthily. I'll be honest, it was great at first! I ate my favourite foods, packed with fat, carbohydrates and sugar.

However, it didn't take long before my body reacted. During these five months I gained two stone and didn't exercise, even though I was working as a personal trainer. My skin got in a terrible state and due to my lack of exercise even an old scuba diving injury returned causing me terrible lower back pain.

Posture is something that can often be overlooked and is frequently the cause of pain and discomfort within our bodies, particularly in our backs. Posture plays a crucial role in how our bodies operate and during these initial five months, mine was abysmal. If you suffer from poor posture or tight muscles too, follow the Myo Clinic Stretch Routine found later in the book, to help target the muscle groups directly.

After just three months of living in this unhealthy way, I found it was also beginning to have an impact on my attitude to life. I felt lethargic, uncomfortable and unable to fit into my clothes with ease. As a result, my self-esteem plummeted to the point where I could no longer get undressed in changing rooms, for fear that people would look at me and judge me. Perhaps they were, and the truth hurts!

But it wasn't only the outside of my body that changed. My cholesterol was getting higher and higher every month as were my glucose levels. This could have been serious as diabetes is ranked as the third largest killer after heart disease and cancer.

With a wealth of experience training individuals from all walks of life, including Hollywood stars and triathletes, I have ensured all my books contain the knowledge and expertise which I have passed on to my clients. Now I can pass that knowledge on to you too.

The good news is that our bodies are built for adapting and overcoming the stresses and strains we put on them. It's never too late to make a difference and even small changes can have a big impact on your life. You now, your body is constantly talking to you. I want you to recognise those early warning signs which tell you your body is not working at its premium. This book will help identify these signals so you can help your body cure itself with the correct nutrition, exercise, cosmetics and lifestyle. You will also discover how to test your body using simple home health testing kits. I gained the two stone to show how you too can lose excess weight with simple changes to your diet, lifestyle and exercise routine. Remember one thing though, you don't need to be skinny to be healthy.

Most of all I hope that you enjoy these books too. It is important to me that these books are personal, to the point and have no gimmicks in the training and eating plans. The pictures throughout the book have had no air brushing – the spots and fatty areas unfortunately were real. To be honest, I wanted to show you the truth about how easily you can change your life, with simple steps, at home on your own and get similar results. Remember, if I can do it, so can you!

Injury and disclaimer

Muscles and injuries are my field of expertise but before you begin any hard and strenuous exercise and home health testing, you should consult your GP for medical reassurance.

When I started my 12-week programme I saw my GP to explain to him what I had planned. Also, I wanted to ensure that home testing kits would give me accurate enough results on which I could base my health and fitness tests.

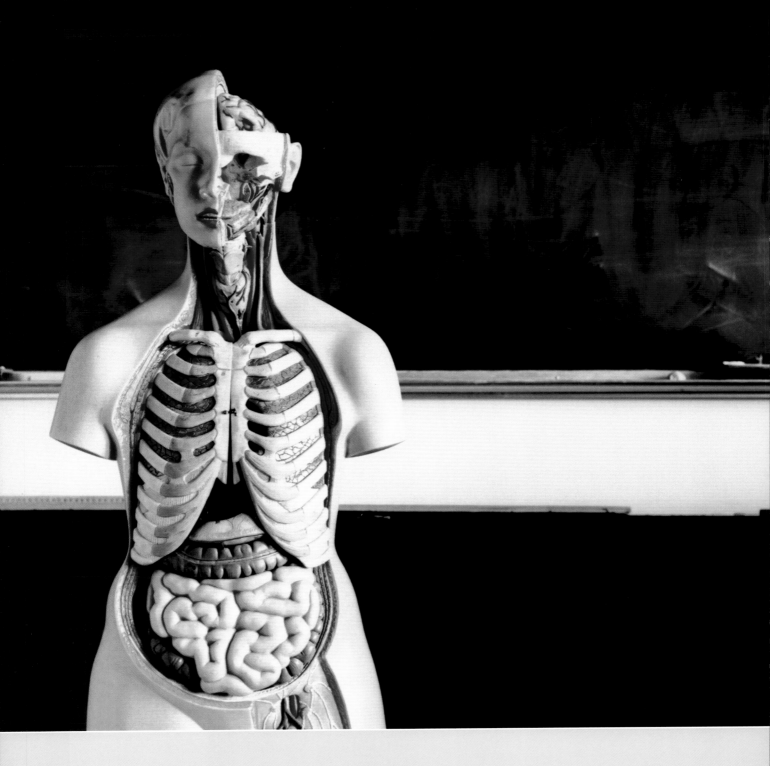

know your body
inside and out

It is important to know your body inside and out. What is normal for you, may not be normal for someone else and vice versa. Everyone can say that they have noticed things about their body which were not normal for them at one time or another. Your body talks to you all the time, perhaps only in subtle measures but by learning to read these signals, it will enable you to act on anything that may be upsetting your well-being or disturbing your equilibrium.

The signs may be small and you may feel that they are even unimportant, like having yellow fingers for example. This could simply be a result of nicotine discoloration, however, it could also be a warning sign for a disorder in your liver or lungs. Try not to take anything for granted.

Knowing how to differentiate between these small signals before they turn into actual symptoms of a disorder, is a delicate matter and should not be rushed. The following information is an easy reference guide to highlight some things that may be troubling you and how you can watch out for signs of poor health in your own body.

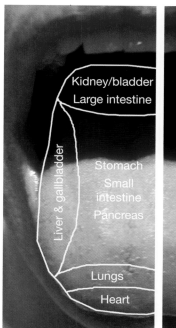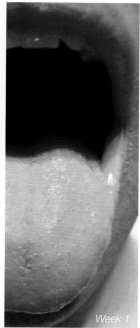

WEEK 1 – please note the teeth marks on the side of my tongue and the slightly red tip. Both of these signs indicate poor nutrition, something that the 12 week nutrition book helped me to alleviate by showing me how to eat a healthy balanced diet.

Tongue

We can detect a lot about the health of a person by looking at aspects of their tongue, such as changes to the shape, size, colour, texture and coating. In fact, the tongue is still used today in Chinese medicine to help diagnose various health concerns. The tongue is covered with several types of papillae or nodules that continually shed and grow like hair, making it a great source of information about our health.

This is a guide for a healthy tongue:

Size and shape
Normal and proportionate to the body

Colour
Salmon or pinky red shade

Texture
Smooth with no marks or cracks

Coating
Thin, white, moist coating across the whole tongue

Here are some things to look out for when investigating your tongue. These could be caused by different conditions or could well be an indication of possible problems within certain body systems. Remember, this is just a guideline.

Size and shape

Big and unusually red
The protective papillae could be being damaged, for example, by teeth or dentures rubbing on the tongue.

Swollen
This could be due to poor digestion. For swollen sides of the tongue, look towards the liver being overworked or a problem within the gallbladder.

Colour

Unusually red

Possibly acute fever. If it is also smooth, it may indicate a vitamin B12 deficiency or an intestinal disorder where nutrients are not being adequately absorbed.

Red tip

Indication of depression, a lack of sleep or stress.

Pale

Possible lack of nutrients within the body such as vitamin B12, folic acid. It may also be caused by a hormone imbalance.

Purple

Poor circulation, poor nutrition or a lack of vitamin B complex and minerals.

Texture

Peeling

Dry mouth or a deficiency in vitamin B.

Teeth marks

Normally occurs with a swollen tongue and could suggest digestion problems.

Scrotal tongue

An indication of an infection or poor nutrition.

Groovy tongue

Something people are usually born with and may not be noticed right away. It tends to become more noticeable as you age.

Coating

White

Indication of the recovery from a recent fever or a poor diet lacking in fibre.

Black

Possible reaction to antibiotics or to stomach medication. Poor oral hygiene, smoking, excessive use of mouthwash, infection, digestion or poorly managed diabetes also may cause this.

Brown and yellow

Trapped bacteria and food or excessive smoking and coffee. Take note: the yellow coating is normally seen with a red tip.

Teeth and gums

We all want those pearly white teeth and healthy gums to give the biggest and best smile imaginable. As a rule, I will usually brush my teeth twice a day. But please note that if you are following the information below, please visit your dentist when it is next convenient.

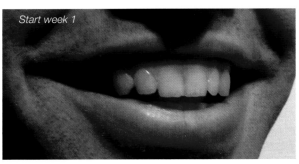

Start week 1

The condition of my teeth and gums remained unchanged throughout my 12 week plan due to my good oral health care.

Here are some things to look out for when investigating your teeth and gums. These could be caused by different conditions or could well be an indication of possible future dental problems, so please consult your dentist if you have any concerns at all.

Teeth

Sensitive

Caused by the thinning of your enamel layer (the outer layer that protects your inner dentine) which causes the dentine underneath to become exposed. Dental erosion, gum recession, gum disease, cracked tooth, tooth fillings and teeth bleaching can all lead to sensitive teeth.

Movement

There is a natural tooth movement that occurs throughout your life. It could be due to a tooth that is about to fall out, trauma, advanced gum disease or, if you are missing a tooth, the teeth on either side can move to fill in that space.

Discoloration

An indication of poor diet like drinking coffee, soft drinks, tobacco, poor dental hygiene, disease, medication, trauma, advanced aging, and choosing the wrong toothpaste could all discolour your teeth.

Gums

Pain

This could be due to an injury, dental disease, tooth decay, scurvy, vitamin B deficiency, iron deficiency, Behcet or Reiter Syndrome.

Swelling

Could be an indication of gum infection, monilia, oral fungal infection, gum disease, gingivitis, poorly fitted dentures, toothpaste or mouthwash allergies. It could also be a possible sign of malnutrition.

Bleeding

This could be due to trauma, disease, mouth sores, systemic conditions, pregnancy and hormonal changes, medication, and vitamin C and K deficiencies.

Lips

Dry and cracked lips could be caused by external factors such as cold weather, or may be a symptom of dehydration or a nutritional deficiency.

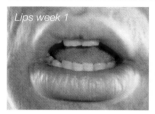
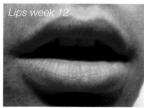

Lips week 1

Lips week 12

You can see on week 1 I had dry and slightly cracked lips but by week 12, I had supple and smooth lips thanks to my new diet and Lush lip balms.

Eyes

Your eyes are a big give-away and say a lot about you, how you are feeling and ultimately how healthy you are. As an organ, the eyes are a great source of information for detecting those early signs of ill health. This is why your doctor will still occasionally examine your eyes when you visit.

Our eyes have more than two million working parts which make them the second most complex organ in your body – the first of course is the brain – and while some say eyes are the windows to the soul others have a more practical view.

Red and/or bloodshot
Small blood vessels in the eyes become inflamed and dilated which causes bloodshot eyes. This may be caused by, or is an indication of, eye strain, fatigue, colds, allergies, ocular rosacea or a deficiency in vitamins B2 and B6 and amino acids commonly found in protein.

It is important to seek medical advice if you are suffering from bloodshot eyes along with any of these symptoms: severe headache, blurred vision, mental confusion, nausea/vomiting or if you are seeing halos around lights. This may be an indication of an attack of acute glaucoma (a sudden increase in eye pressure).

Yellow eye
If the whites of your eyes turn yellow it could be a possible indication of a liver problem such as jaundice, gallbladder concerns, Gilbert's syndrome, sickle cell anaemia, pancreatic cancer or yellow fever.

Dry eyes
This condition occurs when the eyes don't produce enough tears to keep them moist. It is very common in women, especially after the menopause, due to the body's reduction of the oestrogen hormone.

This could also be environmental, for example, due to windy, dry or hot air or air conditioning. Also a sluggish thyroid, constant contact lens usage, a deficiency in omega 3 and 6 or a reaction to prescriptive and non-prescriptive drugs could also cause dry eyes.

Watery eyes
Too many tears being produced could be linked to allergies, a deficiency in vitamin B2 or ocular rosacea.

Bags under the eyes
Puffy pouches of skin under the eye. This is common as the skin around the eye ages and loses elasticity. Depression, insomnia or deprived sleep, crying, a high level of salt intake, a sluggish thyroid, fluid retention, kidney problem or a bad reaction to medicine can encourage bags under the eye area.

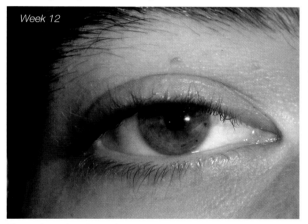

Week 12

Throughout the 12 weeks, my eyes were only effected a couple of times from tiredness, which caused bags under my eyes.

Circles under the eyes
These could be indications of sleep deprivation, digestive problems, sluggish liver, eczema or allergies.

Bulging eyes
Possibly due to an overactive thyroid. It is important to visit your doctor if you suspect this.

Yellowish lump / bump on the cornea
If you notice these small yellow lumps, don't worry, they tend to be age spots called Pinguecula.

Spots on the eye
Red spots on the whites of your eyes are usually blood vessels which have burst. It is normally caused by forceful sneezing or coughing, injury or high blood pressure.

Nails

Your fingernails and toenails actually count as part of your skin and are another great way of highlighting a number of medical and nutritional conditions. Nails are made of protein (keratin) and contain less water than skin, which makes them harder and protects the ends of fingers and toes.

Fingernails take around four months to grow out, while toenails take at least six. If your nail growth is slower than average, it is possible that you may have a fungal infection or a nutritional deficiency like a lack of iron perhaps.

This is a guide for healthy nails.

Texture
Smooth, no ridges, thickness or cracks

Shape
No exaggerated curving up or down at the ends

Nail bed colour
Pink

Colour of nails
White

Here are some things to look out for when investigating your nails.

Texture

Horizontal ridges
These go from side to side across your nail and can be an indication of a thyroid concern, stress, vitamin B deficiency or the result of a nail injury that has stunted nail growth.

Vertical ridges
These go from the nail bed up to the tip. They may be due to nutritional disorders, a lack of iron or a kidney disorder.

Pitted nails
This could be caused by lack of vitamin C, psoriasis, deficiency in protein and is a common sign for autoimmune disorders.

Thick nails
Could be a result of poor circulation, injury, fungal infection, poor diet or diabetes.

Rough nails
If they have a sandpaper type texture, rough nails could indicate a skin or hair disorder such as psoriasis or eczema.

Brittle or cracked nails
Often this is due to the use of harsh cleaning products, a thyroid disease, iron deficiency, vitamin A deficiency or a lack of calcium.

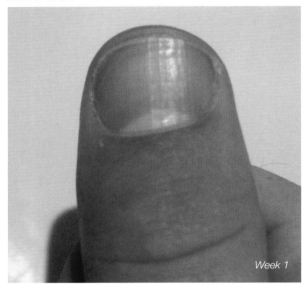

Week 1

Looking at my thumb nail from week 1, you will notice that I have vertical ridges across the nail and a horizontal ridge at the top. This indicates nutritional deficiency.

Shape

Nails curve upwards (resembles a spoon)
Possible nutritional deficiency, a lack of iron or a vitamin B12 deficiency.

Nails curve downwards (clubbed nails)
Could be an indication of bowel disease, liver disease or a lack of oxygen in the body. Once this condition occurs, it is normally permanent.

Nail bed colour

Blue – May be caused by a lung disorder.

Yellow – Sign of a heavy smoker, jaundice or Yellow Nail Syndrome (this is a rare condition however).

Pale – Possible sign of anaemia.

White spots
May be due to nail separation from the nail bed, nail warts, zinc or calcium deficiency, systematic conditions which affects the skin, lungs and other organs.

Hair and scalp

Our hair defines the overall health of a person like no other part of the body. You could say that our luscious locks are a barometer of our general health. Hair condition is a true reflection of the nutrition it receives from the scalp – so the better the diet, the better the hair condition.

Hair is made up from protein (keratin) and minerals which go through the hair growth cycle. The hair has a growth phase followed by a resting phase then a shedding phase. It then repeats the cycle.

When we look at hair, we are looking at its condition, texture and volume to gauge how well our bodies are nourished.

Here are some things to look out for when investigating your hair.

Condition

Dry scalp
This could be due to the environment, hard water, poor diet or the improper use of hair products.

Flaky scalp / dandruff
Dandruff is not contagious and is not usually a serious problem. Some cases of excessive dandruff with intense itching and patches of flaky skin elsewhere on your body are most likely a form of eczema.

A flaky scalp may be caused by or is an indication of a fungus (malassezia), hormone changes, stress, neurological disorders, infrequent shampooing, skin ailments (psoriasis or infections) or the improper use of hair products.

Brittle and split ends
Again these could be due to the environment, a poor diet, lack of protein and essential fatty acids, thyroid disease, menopause, excessive washing and drying, using bleaching and dye products, iodine deficiency, pregnancy or the improper use of hair products.

Volume

Thinning / hair loss
This is normally determined by our genes and the ageing process, but may also be caused by a poor diet, lack of iron or possible thyroid disease.

Texture

Dry
This can be an indication of a poor diet, the environment, lack of protein and essential fatty acids, thyroid disease, menopause, excessive washing and drying, using bleaching and dye products, iodine deficiency, pregnancy or the improper use of hair products.

Greasy/oily
Greasy hair occurs due to an overproduction of sebum, a waxy substance from the sebaceous glands, which keeps the hair supple, soft and waterproof. Fine hair tends to be greasier due to having more sebaceous glands. It may also be caused by genetics, the improper use of hair products or a lack of regular hair cleaning.

Skin

Our skin is a reliable indicator for assessing general health as it is quite obvious when a person is run down, tired or ill by simply looking at their skin. Just think of all those skin creams and serums produced and marketed to millions of people across the world, claiming to dispel aged or tired looking skin! Really, a good routine and a healthy balance is the basis for picture perfect skin.

Our skin protects us from the environment, provides a unique barrier to infection and helps excrete waste and toxins from within the body. It regulates and maintains a healthy balance of fluids and minerals and is of course the source of our sensory receptors for touch. It is the largest organ of the body and is indirectly linked to almost every part of your body, except the eyes and teeth.

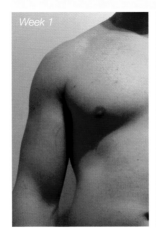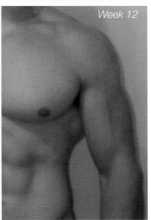

Week 1 *Week 12*

Look closely and in the picture on the left you will see a breakout on my chest. But in the next you can see an amazing difference in my skin condition and physique.

Here are some things to look out for when investigating your skin.

Colour

Pale

Could be an indication of anaemia or iron deficiency.

Blue tone

May be caused by oxygen deficiency in the blood, exposure to cold temperature, lung disease or heart disease.

Yellow tone

Jaundice, the consumption of too much beta-carotene (foods such as carrots) or too much vitamin A.

Gray tone

Excessive smoking, a sluggish liver, cardiovascular disease or feeling unwell.

Red tone

Rosacea, over exertion, inflammation or burns can contribute to a red skin tone. Caught in the early stages, rosacea may cause flushing or blushing, but can progress to permanent redness. The rash consists of tint pimples as well as dilated blood vessels under the skin and may be found on the face and body, which can cause an itching and burning sensation.

Texture

Dark patches on the skin

Possible indication of diabetes and insulin resistance, a hormonal disorder or an adrenal gland concern can form these patches.

Scaly rash

This can be an indication of psoriasis, an infection or emotional stress.

It is common to find random lumps and bumps either on top or beneath the skin surface from time to time and most of these are harmless. Some however are not. If you notice a change in the size or shape of a lump or bump do not hesitate to see your doctor. Early detection of any pre-cancerous or cancerous cells will help treatment. Listen to your body.

Facial skin

We get oily and dry skin on both our body and face. Here are some things to look out for when investigating your facial skin more closely.

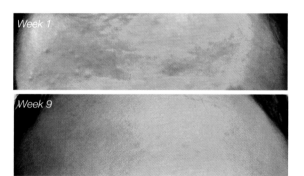

Look at the amazing difference 12 weeks can make to your skin with the right nutrition, cosmetics and advice. Refer to the Lush section for the facial products which helped to clear up the spot breakout on my forehead.

Colour

Rosy cheeks

These can be due to a hot flush, over exertion, rosacea, sun damage or an autoimmune inflammation disease.

Dark patches

These can result from pregnancy, sun damage, a reaction to medication or contraceptive pill or indicate high levels of oestrogen.

Texture

Oily/greasy

The reason for oily or greasy skin is overproduction of sebum, a waxy substance from the sebaceous glands. This could be an indication of stress, pregnancy, hormone imbalance, medication, genetics, poor diet (high sodium intake, sugar and saturated fat). The improper use of cosmetic products or a deficiency in vitamin B2 could also cause an outbreak.

It is not all bad news, your natural sebum slows down the signs of aging!

It is important to highlight the difference between dry skin and dehydrated skin.

Dry skin

This lacks oils and moisture to keep skin supple and regulated. If your face never shows an oily shine and you've never even had a pimple let alone acne, you are most likely to have normal to dry skin.

Dry skin may be caused by genetics, or you may be deficient in essential fatty acids (omega 3, 6 and 9) and/or vitamins A and B. Hormones, skin disorders such as eczema and the improper use of cosmetic products or the environment could also dry your skin.

Dehydrated skin

This is caused by the lack of water within the cells of the skin. If you have had visible pores, especially around your chin, nose or eyebrows and are prone to spots but your skin has a dry and scaly appearance, you probably have dehydrated skin. It could be due to dehydration throughout your body, skin disorders (eczema), the improper use of cosmetic products or the environment.

Combination skin

This is characterised by oily patches in certain areas and dry/dehydrated areas in other parts of your face. The normal areas for the oily patch are known as the T-zone: the forehead, nose, cheeks and the chin. This is due to these areas having more sebaceous glands than other areas of the face, like the eyes and jaw line.

With this combination skin type, awareness must be given to the cosmetic products that you use so that you do not aggravate the problem areas further.

Sensitive skin

Thin or fine textured skin reacts quickly to the heat and cold temperatures and so is easily affected by the environment (sun burn and wind chills).This skin type is usually dry and delicate which is prone to allergic reactions. Again, awareness must be given to the cosmetic products you use so as to not irritate the skin.

With all of the information you have just gained, you may now be wondering, what can you do to help yourself.

One thing you may have noticed is that poor nutrition, lacking in vitamins and minerals plays a large factor in your body's signs for poor health. By changing the way you eat and by choosing a diet rounded, nutritious and high in vitamins and minerals, your body will return to its full health. You will be able to achieve the rounded diet by following the *Train to Become Nutrition Book.*

For any health concerns that you may have, you can help yourself in many ways, ranging from homeopathic remedies and supplements to holistic therapies. Whatever concerns you may have, remember there is nothing too big or too small for your GP. They are there to help you.

Skin care cycle

There are a lot of things you can do to keep your skin healthy, feeling fresh, soft and looking young. Maintaining a healthy diet, getting enough exercise, staying hydrated, avoiding any sun damage to the skin and having low stress levels are all things that aid in keeping skin healthy. The skin care cycle has three main steps which should be followed daily to ensure a truly glowing complexion:

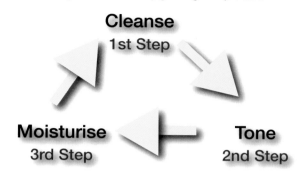

What is cleansing?

Throughout the day your skin is exposed to all kinds of things which clog up your pores such as exhaust fumes, pollution, bacteria and dirt. Your skin naturally looses dead cells, excretes sweat (laced with toxins which your body is pushing out) and excess sebum.

By the end of the day, all this grime lies on the top of the skin and needs removing. When you cleanse, you remove this build-up. Oil based, clay and scrub cleansers will also remove the top layer of dead skin.

What is toning?

This step is so simple and so often overlooked. Ultimately it is crucial to balance the skin, add nutrients and increase hydration. Toning removes any remaining grime left by the cleanser (which is especially important with oil based cleansers) and will balance the pH of the skin. It will also aid in the tightening of pores and helps the skin absorb oils more effectively.

What is moisturising?

This is the most important step in the cycle and helps keep skin young and soft. Think about a piece of leather for example. Adding oil keeps it from drying out, losing vibrancy and wrinkling. Cleansing removes the skin's natural oils on dry skin, on oily skin it signals to the skin to stimulate more oil production often causing over production. By not replacing these oils, the skin must work harder to balance itself.

A moisturiser is not just oil though, it should be a blend of good quality ingredients as it sinks into the skin. Using a cheaper alternative often means cheaper ingredients that will have a long term negative effect on the skin's appearance.

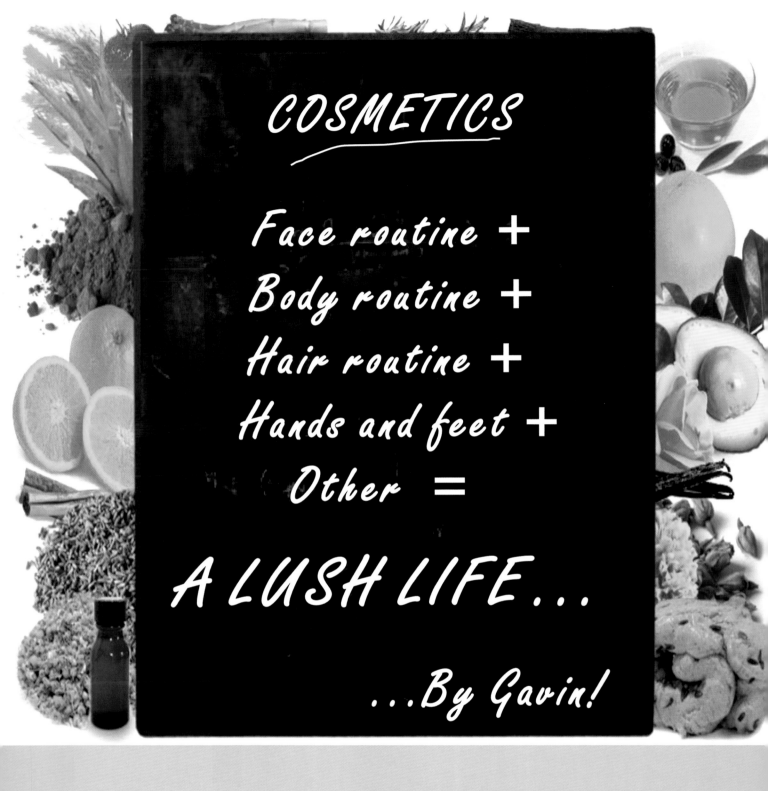

COSMETICS

Face routine **+**
Body routine **+**
Hair routine **+**
Hands and feet **+**
Other **=**

A LUSH LIFE...

...By Gavin!

revitalise your body
back to health

It is uncommon to find anyone who has skin or hair with a perfect balance of oils and nutrients. It tends to be either excessively oily skin or simple dry skin, while people with dry skin probably have dry hair too. If you have read the **know your body inside and out** chapter, you will have noticed that nutrition plays an important role in the health of our hair and skin – as well as the cosmetics we use. *The Train to Become Nutrition Book* will guide you through the 12-week healthy eating plan to balance your body and bring it up to its healthy potential. However the use of cosmetic products shouldn't be overlooked and did indeed help counteract my body's problems.

Cosmetics

There are hundreds of products aimed at consumers, proclaiming how they can stop the signs of ageing or take away those dark circles from beneath your eyes. We fall for the slogans in the advertising campaigns and buy the product and, more often than not, we are unhappy with the results. But do we pay attention to the chemicals and oils that are in these potions and lotions and to the harmful effects that these have on our skin?

I asked myself this question and began looking at the varying products and companies available and became hopelessly confused and frustrated by it all! I had begun to ask the same questions about buying cosmetics as I would ask when buying food: is it local, fresh, organic with no preservatives and, above all, is it value for money?

I continued my research and then it hit me – it had been in front of me all of the time! My friend, Simon Constantine, is involved with the handmade and ethical cosmetic company, **Lush** cosmetics! The more I found out about Lush, the more I became sure that this company would have everything that I was looking for in healthy skin and body care products.

All of the products are natural and hand-made. And, when I first visited my local Lush shop the staff in the stores were incredibly helpful. I explained the 12-week fitness and health plan that I was about to undertake and they were able to show me where I was going wrong with the cosmetics and creams I was using. They recommended products to me that were specifically designed for my skin concerns so that I could better pursue my quest to becoming healthy.

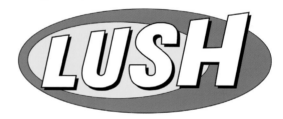

A Lush life. Just so you know, Lush believe in making effective products from fresh organic fruit and vegetables, the finest essential oils and safe synthetics.

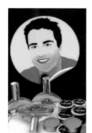

Here is a little something about Lush by my friend Simon Constantine, *Lush Head of Buying.*

'We buy ingredients only from companies that do not commission tests on animals – we test our products on humans. We invent our own products and fragrances and make them fresh by hand using little or no preservatives or packing. We use only vegetarian ingredients and tell you exactly when the products are made.

'Cosmetics these days can often be heavily preserved and have minimum amounts of good quality ingredients. The best way to do this is to educate yourself and to make discerning purchases of products. Three for two offers are attractive but buying the right product for you is much more important and is better for you.

'At Lush, we use natural ingredients as we believe they provide the best and most effective way of helping the skin, whatever its needs are. We use 8000 bunches of flowers and 50 tonnes of fresh fruit and vegetables in our products each year in the UK alone. From English honey for its antiseptic and healing properties, through to lavender oils for their therapeutic and calming aromas – it's always our first choice to use a natural ingredient.

'One of Lush's founding principles is one of fresh product – the quicker we make and sell our products to you, then the less we have to worry about throwing in preservatives and other nasties. For us preservatives are unnecessary if we can make the product right, we now have 71% of our products preservative free. Sometimes we re-invent classic products so they require no preservative at all such as our solid products ranges, shampoos, soaps and ballistics.

'We produce as near to our shops as possible. In the UK we have our factory in Dorset where our products are all handmade. Making our products by hand means we can have the artisan feel to our product creation that we feel a machine just wouldn't give you.

Although we don't like to brag, at Lush we have had some wonderful feedback from customers over the years who have been very satisfied with our products. Gavin has quoted some of these comments relating to the Lush products that he used during his 12-week plan.'

Below is a list of the Lush products I used to get my skin and body back into great shape over the 12-week plan.

For the face

Follow Lush's four simple steps to help you revitalise your face to perfection:

1st step   cleanse
2nd step   mask (once a week)
3rd step   tone
4th step   moisturise

If an exfoliant cream is needed, you'll find them in the cleanser or the fresh face masks section. You should exfoliate after you have cleansed your face, to help get rid of those extra dead skin cells to leave your face glowing and radiant.

My skin care

I can finally say goodbye to my spots thanks to following this Lush skin routine:

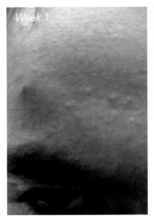
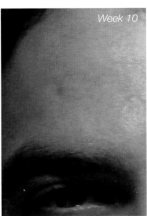

As you can see, I suffered badly with spots from a poor diet and little knowledge of skin care. Week 12 shows a complete transformation both with my skin which you can see and with my confidence which you can't.

Fresh Farmacy

This is an amazing cleanser and most effective for troubled skin as it helped clear my spots using ingredients with calming properties such as chamomile, rose, tea tree and lavender.

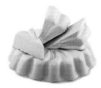

Angels of Bare Skin

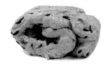

I used this every three days as another cleanser. It helped soothe, balance, soften and calm the skin as well as being slightly exfoliating.

Tea Tree Water

This is a toner, which I used to detoxify and to stimulate my skin with grapefruit, tea tree and refreshing juniper berry.

Enzymion

This face moisturiser helped my oily prone skin with its ingredients containing natural acids from organic fruit which break down oils before making the skin shine.

Grease lightning

I used this as a spot gel to get rid of the redness and to calm down my outbreaks. Simply the best. I highly recommend this product!

Face mask

Cosmetic Warrior

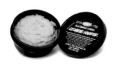

I used this once every three weeks for the first six weeks. It is an antibacterial mask which helped to combat my spots.

Love Lettuce

I used this mask for the remaining six weeks to exfoliate, brighten and nourish my skin.

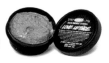

Once my skin was back to what was normal for me (which took around four weeks) I introduced some new products into my skincare regime:

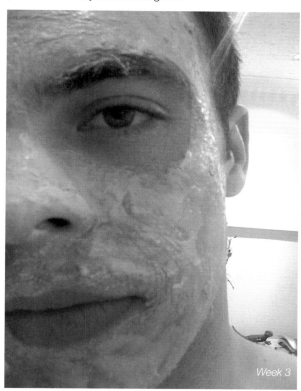

Week 3

This was the very first face mask I used from Lush. It worked really well afterwards, helping reduce my spots – but I think I have a small resemblance to a troll!

Coalface

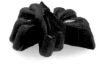

This is a cleanser to keep oily skin balanced. It is gentle and will not dry the skin as much as Fresh Farmacy can.

Breath of Fresh Air

This toner refreshed and hydrated my skin.

Vanishing Cream

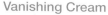
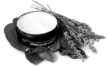

This very light face moisturiser really helped make me feel as though I had treated the face without making it feel at all oily.

Use the following tables to guide you into choosing the right Lush product for your own hair and skin types. These tables are only a guideline as all Lush products have many properties in them to suit all different conditions that may not be listed. I would recommend that once you know what you're looking for, you speak to one of the helpful Lush staff who will help guide you in the right direction.

1st step: Cleansers

Keep these in your arsenal to combat dirt and grime:

	Sensitive	Dry	Dehydrated	Oily	Combination	Exfoliator
Angels on Bare Skin	✓	✓	✓	✓	✓	✓
Aqua Marina	✓					
Baby Face*		✓	✓			
Coalface				✓		✓
Dark Angels				✓	✓	✓
Fresh Farmacy				✓		
Herbalism				✓	✓	✓
Mask of Magnaminty				✓	✓	✓
Ocean Salt				✓	✓	
Ultrabland*	✓	✓	✓	✓	✓	

Comments from Lush's customers:

Ultrabland

'This stuff is a miracle worker! You can use it for pretty much anything! Works wonders on removing make up (even waterproof mascara), moisturising, soothing cracked skin, lip balm, conditioning nails... you name it, it can probably do it! I use it to sooth my son's eczema after a bath – works a treat!'

Baby Face

'What a delightful butter bar, it melts on my skin to remove the dirt on my face and puts back moisture. It's also fabulous for my make-up removal and its scent makes you feel an everlasting beauty!'

2nd step: Face masks (once a week)

	Sensitive	Dry	Dehydrated	Oily	Combination	Mature	Breakouts	Exfoliator
A Crash Course in Skincare*			✓					
Ayesha						✓		
BB Seaweed	✓	✓	✓		✓			
Brazened Honey				✓				✓
Catastrophe cosmetics	✓				✓		✓	
Cosmetic Warrior				✓			✓	
Cupcake*				✓	✓		✓	
Love Lettuce				✓	✓			✓
Oatifix Fresh Face Mask		✓	✓				✓	✓
The Sacred Truth						✓		

Comments from Lush's customers*:

A Crash Course

'Love this, it made my skin so calm and even, It smells delicious as well. Calmed my spots right down :)'

Cupcake

'This is perfect for my troubled teenaged and oily skin. It removed my excess oil and calmed down my spot breakouts. Like indulging in a chocolate bar, but much better for your skin!'

3rd step: Toners

	Sensitive	Dry	Dehydrated	Oily	Combination
Breathe of Fresh Air	✓	✓	✓		
Eau-Roma Water*	✓	✓	✓		✓
Etc Etc	✓	✓	✓	✓	✓
Tea Tree Water*				✓	
Tea Tree Tab				✓	
Vit C Tab			✓	✓	✓
Vit E Tab	✓	✓	✓		

Comments from Lush's customers*:

Eau-Roma Water

'I use this and I don't have dry / sensitive skin. It's nice and refreshing and isn't too strong. It's perfect for my combination skin. Doesn't dry my skin out and removes excess oil. It's definitely a great product :)'

Tea Tree Water

'I have problem skin and I have been using this daily for the past week or so and can definitely see the difference, my skin looks great again and the spots have almost gone!'

4th step: Moisturisers

	Sensitive	Dry	Dehydrated	Oily	Combination	Mature
Celestial	✓	✓				
Cosmetic Lad		✓	✓		✓	
Enzymion				✓		
Gorgeous	✓	✓	✓		✓	✓
Imperialis	✓	✓	✓	✓	✓	
Paradise Regained		✓	✓			✓
Skin Drink*		✓	✓			
Skin Nanny		✓				✓
Skin's Shangri La			✓			✓
Vanishing Cream	✓			✓	✓	

Comments from Lush's customers*:

Skin Drink

'I'd resigned myself to never finding a moisturiser that actually moisturised my dry skin and didn't cause it to flare up in a rash, after years of trying pretty much everything, Skin Drink came to the rescue. I love it! Thanks Lush! X'

Enchanted Eye Cream

'I'm 47, and have used PLENTY of eye creams, and this is the best I've found to date. It works quickly – I've noticed results in less than a week! It also helps the "frown line" between my eyes! This combined with Skin's Shangri La is a winning ticket for the over 40's!'

For the body

Follow Lush's three simple steps for regaining and maintaining great skin condition:

1st step   wash
2nd step   scrub
3rd step   moisturise

I used two different shower routines and one bath routine. The shower routines were based on time and the general shower routine I had was mostly after training with just the first step – cleansing. Whereas the luxurious routine I had before bed with all three steps. The bath routine was for those special days when I had more time to relax.

My general shower routines

Quick shower alternating the liquid shower products and using the scrub if I had time:

1st step

Happy Hippy – gave me gentle but a great pick me up!

Flying Fox – had a soothing and calming effect on my skin

The Olive Branch – balanced and soothed my skin changes as well as smelling great.

2nd step

Rub Rub Rub – rejuvenated and revitalised my skin.

Buffy – helped exfoliate and soften my skin and prevented any ingrown hairs due to shaving.

My luxuriously long shower routine:

1st step

The Olive Branch – balanced and soothed my skin changes as well as smelling great.
Happy Hippy or Flying Fox

2nd step

Buffy – helped exfoliate and soften my skin and prevented any ingrown hairs due to shaving or **Rub Rub Rub**

Foot scrub

Running to the Embassy – this clever bar scrubbed, moisturised and conditioned my feet in one.

3rd step

Dream Cream – I used this all over especially after shaving or **Ultralight**

Foot moisturiser

Fair Trade Foot Lotion – I used this after every luxury shower to completely moisturise my feet. I feel this foot lotion helped to eradicated my athletes' foot.

My bath routine

During the 12 week health and fitness plan, I had a bath every Saturday night or Sunday morning and relaxed with Lush bath products as I was shaving my body.

I used most of the bath ballistics, melts and bars. All of the bath products are down to personal preference but my favourite bath ballistic is Vanilla Mountain because of the smell, Blue Skies bubble bar because it turns the bath lovely and blue and Ceridwyn's Cauldron which is the best one of all, you just have to try it!

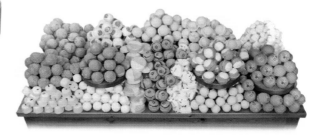

Lush have a huge selection of bath products. You have to try a bath ballistic, they smell amazing.

Comments from Lush's customers*:

Sex Bomb

'Simply made me feel like a goddess with the use of aphrodisiac essential oils, is the perfect preparation for that quiet night in with my boyfriend...'

Floating Island Bath Melt

'This is the best bath melt product ever. It leaves your skin so smooth and gives a relaxing feel to the body. Would recommend it to anyone who is stressed and needs a helping lift to relax.'

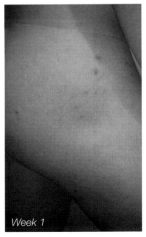
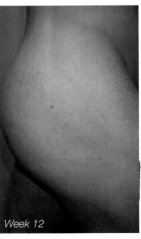

Week 1 *Week 12*

I have to admit that I had a poor lifestyle. I sat around, a lot like a couch potato not realising that I was getting a spotty posterior. By week 12, I had changed my lifestyle and, by being really active and with a little helping hand from Lush, I changed my body condition inside and out.

For the hair

It is as important to condition your hair as it is to wash it. Lush have a great variety of hair products that suit all types of hair conditions. My hair is very fine and has a tendency to be greasy so Lush staff prescribed me the following products to use.

I Love Juicy

It's fantastic on my oily prone hair. It smells great and gave back some volume to my thinning hair as well as normal shine instead of a greasy shine.

Veganese

This balanced and conditioned my hair after shampooing and made my hair feel silky smooth with a nice natural shine.

King of the Mods

What an excellent soft-hold gel. It smells like sherbet sweets!

I Love Juicy

'If you wash your hair daily only to find it's oily again by midday then you MUST try this! I still wash daily – though I could probably leave it a day – but my hair looks clean right up until I next shower. It's made it very shiny & soft too, seems to help keep it straight & the sweet fruity smell stays all day! ...Plus I'm using 1/4 of the amount I did with 'normal' shampoo... Goes well with Veganese."

Veganese

'Lovely :) when smelling it out of the bottle, it seemed to have very little scent, but once I started applying it, I found out it had a lovely fragrance to it which remained in my hair after rinsing! :) left my hair very soft and tangle free too :) would definitely recommend it :)'

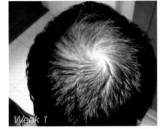
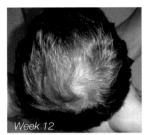

Week 1 *Week 12*

Looking at the week 1 you will see how shiny and greasy my hair was even though it was freshly washed. This is quite unfortunate for me as it makes my balding patch stand out! In comparison, I have more volume and natural shine in the photo on week 12 which I think helps to hide my bald spot – pretty good hey!

I have picked out some shampoos and conditioners for you to choose the right Lush product to suit your hair.

Shampoo

	Oily	Dry	Processed hair	Scalp conditions	Volume	Curly hair
Big*					✓	
Curly Wirly		✓			✓	✓
Cynthia Sylvia Stout		✓			✓	
Godiva		✓			✓	
I love Juicy*	✓				✓	
Jumping Juniper	✓					
Karma Komba		✓		✓		
New Shampoo Bar		✓		✓	✓	
Squeaky Green	✓	✓		✓		
Rehab*		✓	✓	✓		

Conditioner

	Oily	Dry	Processed hair	Scalp conditions	Volume	Curly hair
American Cream	✓	✓	✓			
Coolaulin		✓	✓	✓		✓
Jungle	✓	✓				
Veganese	✓			✓	✓	

Comments from Lush's customers*:

Big

'It is so worth the money. It makes my hair indescribably soft and gives it so much volume, it really is that effective!'

Rehab

'This is without doubt one of the best shampoos that I have ever tried. My hair has been dyed blonde for years and unless I use tons of conditioner on my hair it ends up like straw. Using this, on the other hand, WOWOWOW!! My hair is soft, shiny and actually feels really clean. Loads of people around me keep asking me if I've had my hair done recently as it looks fantastic. I've let a few of my friends try it out for themselves and they absolutely love it...Best ever shampoo...without a doubt.'

For the hands and feet

We use our hands and feet every day without realising and we take them for granted. In my line of work I know that it is very important to keep my hands in good condition. However, I find it very easy to forget about my feet. After the fattening up process I noticed that I had athletes' foot and trench foot through neglect. After using Lush products, even with training almost every day, the difference was amazing.

Hands

Lemon Flutter

I thought this is best just before you go to bed at night time. It helped prevent calluses caused by weight lifting.

Helping Hands

A little help for you hands with this hand cream that is a miracle worker at softening them.

Feet

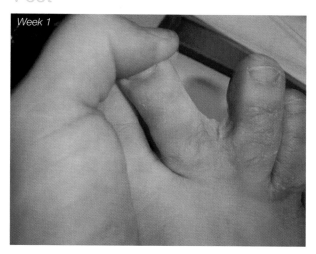

Week 1

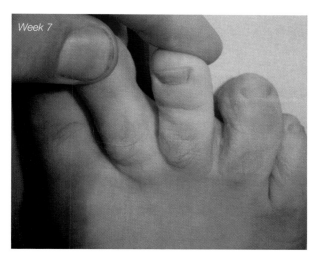

Week 7

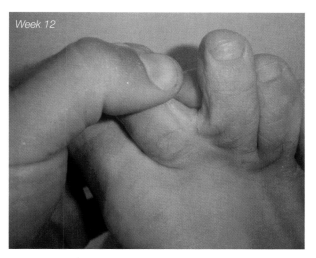

Week 12

I know the beginning picture is not very pretty to look at with a case of athletes' foot but it is quite common in a lot of people. By week seven most of it had cleared up and the itchiness had gone and by week 12, I finally had normal feet. I would say most of this was due to Fair Trade Foot Lotion.

Running to the Embassy

This kept my feet smelling fresh and with natural antibacterial ingredients helped prevent and combat my athletes' foot and trench foot.

Fair Trade Foot Lotion

I used this after I showered to keep my feet smelling fresh and moisturised. In my eyes this was one of the major factors in getting rid of my athletes' foot.

T for Toes

This is a foot deodorant which helped reduce sweat on my feet whilst training, in turn helping to prevent fungal infections.

Volcano

This foot mask helped soften the hard skin on my heels thanks to the papaya fruit ingredient which also encourages cell regeneration. It left my feet really soft and almost as new!

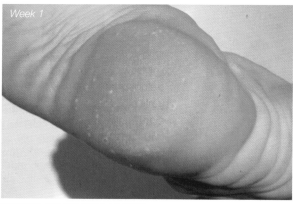
Week 1

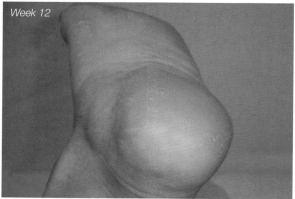
Week 12

This shows my trench foot on week 1 and by week 12, with a little t.l.c., my feet were transformed even though I was running and training all the time.

Handy Gurugu

'Great for eczema. Also keeps my nails hard and strong. It prevents them from breaking and going soft from my daily swimming.'

Pied De Pepper

'Definitely a foot cream for the winter months. Smells delicious and does a very good job of making sore feet happy again. Perfect before bedtime with some fluffy socks, warm PJ's and a mug of hot chocolate! Will definitely use again and again.'

Other routines

You have already seen the amazing change in my lips from week 1 to 12 in the first chapter **know your body inside and out** and Lip Service lip balm is the reason for this improvement.

I suffered a lot of discomfort after shaving my body every week which I did for the purpose of taking these photographs. I felt it would help readers see the weekly changes. The main shaving product I used was Ambrosia.

Lips

Lip Service

This lip balm keeps lips soft and flexible. I used it daily throughout the 12-week plan and I still use it now.

None of your Beeswax

This lip balm is extremely moisturising and tastes of lemon meringue pie!

Honey Trap

'Really good for dry lips. And lasts a long time seeing as I like to top up my balm about 10 times a day! Worth a try!'

Whipstick

'Love it! Makes my lips super smooth and soft. Lovely chocolate smell!'

Shaving

Ambrosia

This is a very gentle product, which I liked to use because I have very sensitive skin and I'm prone to getting a shaving rash. As you can see from my pictures I need to use a good shaving cream for all of the hair I have!

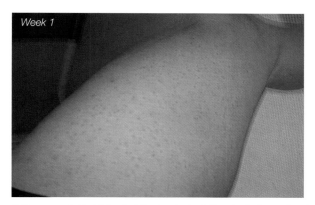

Week 1

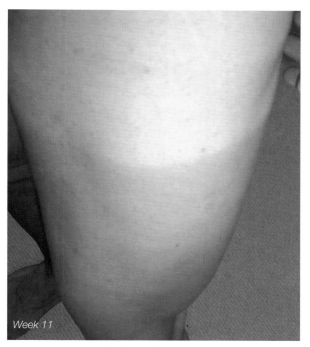

Week 11

All I can say is that it hurt at the beginning! Eventually through using some Lush products like Dream Cream and my due to body getting used to shaving, everything calmed down – even with the sunburn. You can see the difference in my irritated skin from week 1 to week 12.

Your Lush routine

Use the table below to note which Lush products you use for each body part. You may also want to note how and when to use each product as this will enable you to monitor the effectiveness in the same way. I was able to pinpoint which products were working the best for me, using this method throughout the 12-week plan:

	Product 1	Product 2	When and how to use
Face			
Cleanser			
Toner			
Mask			
Moisturiser			
Body			
Shower gel			
Exfoliator			
Moisturising			
Bath ballistics			
Hair			
Shampoo			
Conditioner			
Hands & feet			
Scrub			
Mask			
Moisturiser			

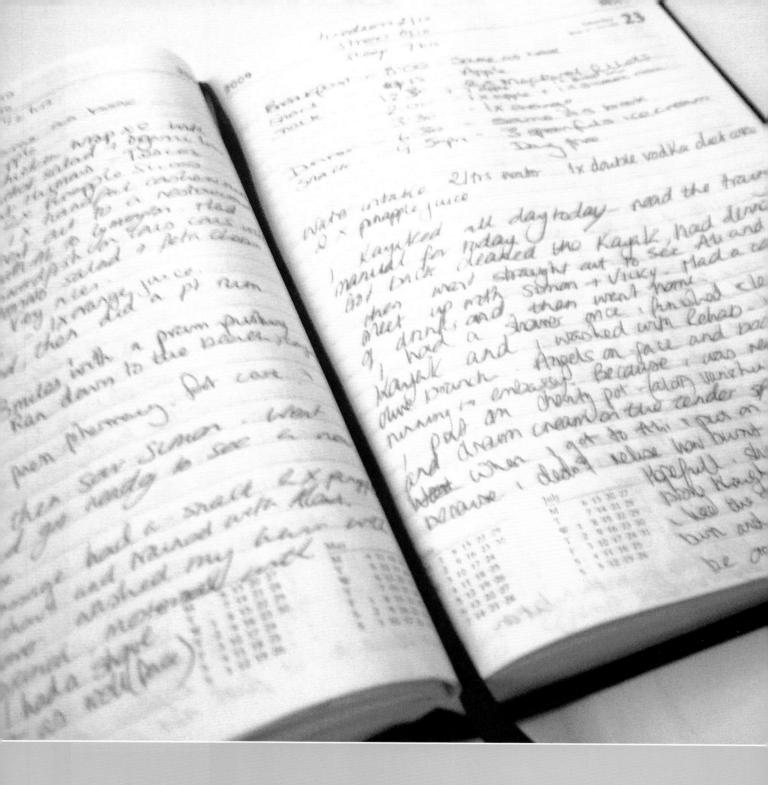

take control
of the basics

When we look at the basics for health, we are looking at the situations that we face everyday of our lives. How we handle stress, how we overcome tiredness and how we get the most out of ourselves. It is these situations that change the way we look at life and make us into who we are. If we can take hold of these basics, we will be able to get more out of ourselves and others.

Stress

We feel stress when pressure is placed upon us, whether actual or imagined. It can be harmful but a certain amount can be good for us to help motivation, performance and productivity. Too much stress however can prompt depression, so please keep a close eye on yourself and others.

People react differently to stress; some have a higher threshold than others. Reasons for stress are very broad and unpredictable. It is a common fact that stress can be caused by demanding deadlines at work, relationship concerns, financial pressures, illness or loss of a loved one. These and many more concerns can cause anxiety and stress which can lead to physical, emotional and mental health problems.

When we are faced with circumstances that are stressful to our mind and body, the body release hormones (chemicals like cortisol, adrenaline), which helps regulate our responses internally.

Adrenaline, for instance, is released to help us cope with dangerous or unexpected conditions. These invoke the flight or fight impulse – the biological response to acute stress.

It is interesting however, that when faced with a situation in which you are prevented from either fleeing or fighting, such as being in a crowded underground tube station, these chemicals are not released.

If you have a build up of these chemicals due to them not being used, the consequences are felt throughout the body such as an increase in blood pressure, heart rate and sweat production.

Stress can cause any single or multiple conditions. The list below is not meant to scare you, it is simply to emphasize the need to try to control and minimise any stress you may feel in your life.

- Heart disease
- Muscular tension
- Pain
- Diet
- Depression
- Weight gain/loss/obesity
- Digestive problems
- Sleep problems
- Autoimmune diseases
- Lower immunity causing more colds, feeling run down, etc
- Raised cholesterol
- Skin complaints

As you can see from these pictures the female was suffering from stress due to her work and lifestyle. We managed to beat the stress and calm down the skin dramatically within a short period by following the steps on the next page.

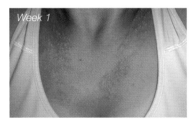

Week 1

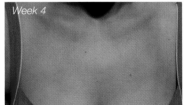

Week 4

Stress responses

Stress affects our bodies in many ways and on many levels. Have a look below to understand your stress responses.

Physiological
Tension from posture or over use.

Emotional
Anger, fear and hate are all reflected in our postures.

Behavioural
Posture imbalance from habit.

Structural
The body and posture will change to meet any stress imposed upon it.

You can follow these steps to help control your own stress levels.

Step 1 – Your stress levels
These are influenced by numerous things. The key is to have the knowledge and power to monitor your own responses and to seek help or advice when something gets a little too much for you to cope with. How you take control is up to you.

Step 2 – Your sense of control
Have confidence with yourself and your ability to perform. Support from friends and family will encourage you to look on the positive side, to share some of your concerns and will act as a buffer for life's stresses, resulting in you feeling less vulnerable.

Step 3 – Your attitude
Try to have a more optimistic outlook. The ability to manage your emotions and bring them back into balance will enable you to become more calm and relaxed.

Step 4 – Your understanding and preparation
Learn from past stresses and try to be prepared for similar future stresses. For example, when I broke my back in a diving accident, I knew it would be a long road to recovery so I rehabilitated slowly and professionally trying not to worry excessively about things. I made a full recovery and have continued diving with no worries.

My stress results

During my 12-week programme I used the RPE scale to rate my stress levels. As you can see from the graph, my stress levels were fairly high at the start but gradually decreased as I started to eat healthily, to exercise and to take control of my body's condition and lifestyle.

RPE (Rating Perceived Exertion)

For Stress

Throughout the 12-week health plan I used the Borg or RPE scale to track my stress levels in my everyday life. The RPE Scale is a simple method of measuring how a person handles stress on their body. The original scale was introduced by Gunnar Borg who rated exertion on a scale of 6 – 20, although many health practitioners now use a revised scale of 0 – 10 developed by the American College of Sports Medicine. RPE can be applied to absolutely anything.

0 – Not stressed at all
1 – Very, very light stress
2 – Very light stress
3 – Fairly light stress
4 – Light amount of stress
5 – Moderately stressed
6 – Fairly stressed
7 – Stressed
8 – Very stressed
9 – Very, very stressed
10 – Stress is severely affecting life

Use the RPE scale above to track your progress in overcoming stress within the *Train to Become Fitness Book*.

See graph of results opposite.

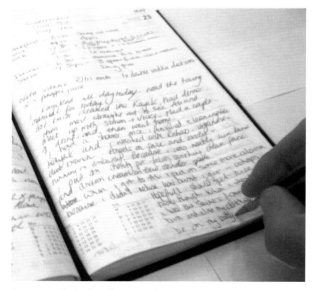

I was caught jotting down my days events and thoughts in my health diary.

OUR STRESS LEVEL RESULTS - MALE & FEMALE

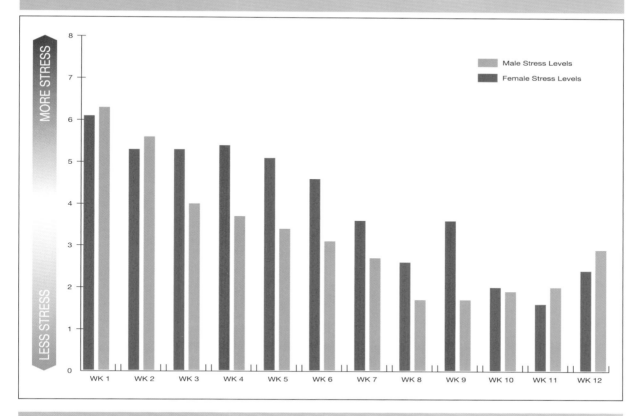

OUR ENERGY LEVEL RESULTS - MALE & FEMALE

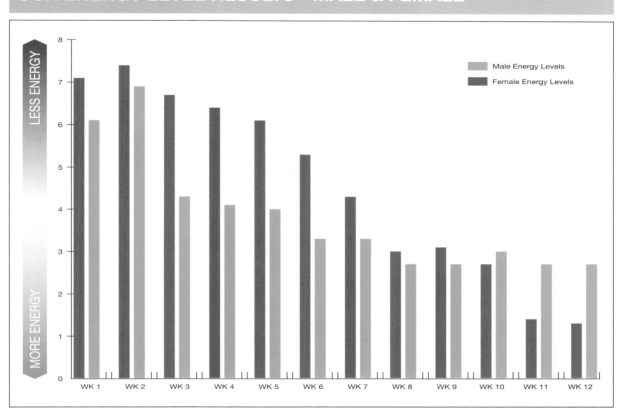

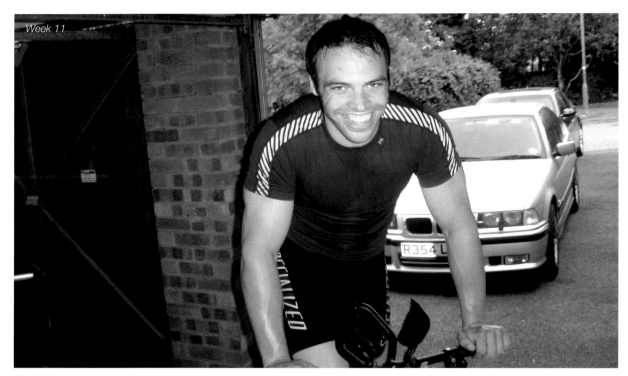

Week 11

I loved all of my training throughout the 12-week fitness programme and you will see from the graph how my energy levels increased as the weeks went by.

Energy levels

It's a fact: having more energy in the body fights fatigue and reduces stress levels. We have all felt tired and lacking in energy from time to time, especially during busy or stressful periods. But if you know the cause then the solution is often easy. More often than not, the reasons are found in our everyday life and habits.

Energy levels can be affected by your diet, how much sleep you get and even your emotional state.

There are so many contributing factors that affect the balance of our emotional and physical state which ultimately affect our energy levels.

You should ask yourself how many of the following items are you managing to help keep your batteries charged:

1. Having regular exercise
2. Drinking plenty of water
3. Eating a balanced diet
4. Sleeping well
5. Controlling stress levels
6. Managing your emotional state

See graph of results on page 25.

Try applying the RPE scale to track your progress in overcoming tiredness within the Train to Become Fitness Book. Simply change the stress levels for a tiredness rating such as:

0 – Not tired at all
1 – Very, very little amount of tiredness
2 – Very little amount of tiredness
3 – Fairly little amount of tiredness
4 – Small amount of tiredness
5 – Moderately tired
6 – Fairly tired
7 – Tired
8 – Very tired
9 – Very, very tired
10 – Too tired to stay awake

My energy level results

On page 25 are my own results which show how I was handling my energy levels on a daily basis. As you can see, my energy levels were fairly high at the start of the 12 weeks but gradually decreased as I started to eat healthily, exercise and basically gain control of my body and its condition. Although I did suffer from a fair amount of tiredness, I was able to manage it by following the same steps.

Behind the scenes...

...it is amazing what good things come from getting fit and healthy. Here I am having a professional photo shoot to promote the Train to Become books in one of the world's leading men's magazines.

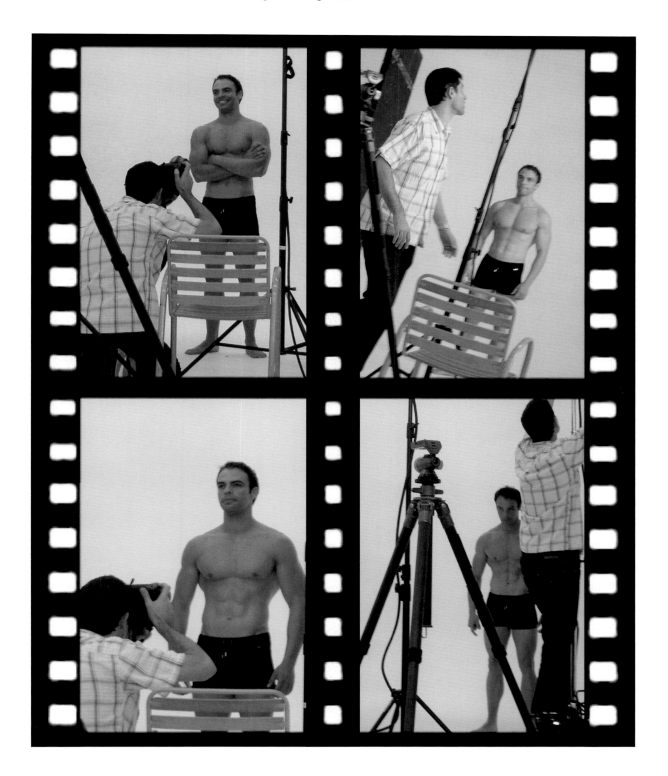

Sleep

Sleep is as important as eating and drinking which is why we spend one third of our lives doing it! It is absolutely vital for maintaining normal levels of cognitive skills including speech, memory, innovative and flexible thinking and it gives the body a chance to recuperate and recover from all of the day's activities.

We all become agitated and stressed when we are tired. The simple and most mundane tasks may become a source of stress due to sleep deprivation. The average amount of sleep needed for adults is around eight hours.

Most adults need around eight hours of sleep on a regular basis to function well, although some require more than others. It is believed the likes of Napoleon, Florence Nightingale and Margaret Thatcher all survived on just four hours sleep a night!

Sleep is triggered by hormones that are active in the brain and respond from cues from the body and the environment. Some of our growth hormones trigger the release of proteins throughout the body to build and repair cells during sleep. Sleep deprivation can prevent this and affect the immune system.

Sleep occurs in a recurrent series of 90 – 110 minutes and is divided into two categories relating to Rapid Eye Movement levels; non-REM sleep and REM sleep which is about 80% of dreamless sleep.

During NREM sleep, your breathing and heart rate slow and blood pressure will be low. This type of sleep is divided into four stages:

Level 1 – Transition between wakefulness to sleep

Level 2 – Makes up 50% of sleep, slowing breathing and heartbeat

Level 3 – Very low respiration and heartbeat

Level 4 – Leads to rapid eye movement sleep known as REM or Level 5

My average amount of sleep per night was six hours, 36 minutes, whilst my female counterpart slept on average seven hours and five minutes per night.

Hydration

Water makes up more than two thirds of the weight in the human body, around 60 – 70% depending on size, shape and the amount of lean tissue (muscle). Muscle consists of approximately 75% water, fat is around 14%, blood has around 82%, and lungs have 90%. Astonishingly, the human brain is made up of 95% water. A mere 2% drop in our body's water supply can trigger signs of dehydration and without water we could die within days.

Water is the most important nutrient for the body. It helps keep your cells, tissues and organs running smoothly, efficiently and effectively. Some of the ways water keeps your body working is by helping to keep it at a constant internal temperature, preventing constipation and it cushions your joints and protects your organs. Fluids are vitally important when you are ill particularly when you lose more water due to fever, diarrhoea or vomiting.

Your body needs a continuous supply of water to stay hydrated. By maintaining an adequate hydration level your body will feel all the more healthy.

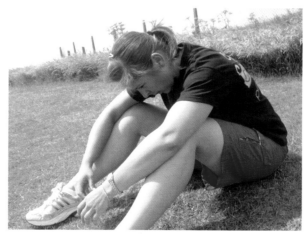

The first week of training was hard both mentally and physically. You can see from this photo after a training session, the female was tired and looking forwards to resting and sleeping. Sleep helps our bodies recover for the next day's activities.

Reasons why water is special:

1. Helps to fight fatigue and tiredness
2. Allows you to exercise, train harder and maintain your strength
3. Is the best detoxing agent available
4. Helps digestion
5. Regulates your metabolism
6. Serves as a lubricant
7. Forms the base for saliva
8. Forms fluids that surround and protect joints
9. Regulates the body temperature as cooling and heating is distributed through perspiration
10. Helps get rid of waste

If you always wait until your mouth is dry to drink water, then you are probably waiting too long and are most likely dehydrated. Dehydration causes a fuzzy, short-term memory, trouble with basic cognitive skills and difficulty focusing on smaller print. Are you having trouble reading this? If so, drink up!

Water comes packaged in different forms so you can have a little variety throughout your day. Did you know that a glass of milk or a serving of juice is actually about 90% water?

Some foods have high water content too such as fruits, vegetables, yogurts and soups. Enjoying these foods regularly can contribute to your water intake and also provide you with many of the vitamins and minerals your body needs.

Here's something to think about:

A common mistake is confusing thirst for hunger so why not drink water if you feel hungry between meals.

How much water is enough?

It is recommended to consume between 1.5 litres – 3 litres a day. During the 12-week plan I drank on average 1.5 litres a day (eight glasses) and that's excluding the fruit drinks, herbal teas and food I consumed. Don't be put off by plain water. Add a cordial to it to make it a little tastier.

A word about fruit drinks

I like to drink fruit juice most mornings. Usually I choose pineapple but that of course is personal preference. The main point to remember when choosing a fruit juice drink is to buy one that is not made from concentrates and is 100% natural, with no added sweeteners or preservatives.

Teas and coffees

As part of the 12-week fitness and nutritional plan, I chose to live a healthy lifestyle which did not cut out any essential dietary needs. I also chose not to completely remove the sociable side of my lifestyle which included alcohol, tea and coffee. I simply chose the healthier option when doing so. For example, when I had a choice between teas or coffees, I chose green tea, herbal tea or decaffeinated tea and coffee. When I was drinking alcohol, I avoided beer and opted for a spirit like vodka with a fruit or diet mixer.

Throughout the 12 weeks I didn't have a coffee, but that is only because I don't have a tendency to drink it normally. Overall I drank three cups of tea with no added sugar and skimmed milk and drank six cups of herbal tea, mainly green tea.

A word about alcohol

During the 12-week plan I had a couple of parties to go to and met up with friends at my local pub. Here is a little advice as to what to choose:

- Spirit with fruit or diet mixer over ales/lager/beer
- Red wine over white wine
- Guinness or ale over beer/lager
- Cider over beer/lager

Here is a rundown of my alcohol intake over the entire 12-week plan. It may sound a lot, but remember, this was over three months:

3 x pints of Guinness
1 x bottle of cider
1 x pint of beer/lager
1 x pint of ale
4 x Vodka (single) and a diet mixer
2 x Vodka (double) and a diet mixer
2 x Malibu and a diet mixer
3 x medium glass of red wine

On average I consumed a little over one alcoholic drink per week.

The average alcohol unit consumption was 2.4 per week – which is the equivalent of having one pint of beer or two single spirits with a diet mixer a week. I didn't actually drink alcohol every week and some of my alcohol consumption was on one occasion.

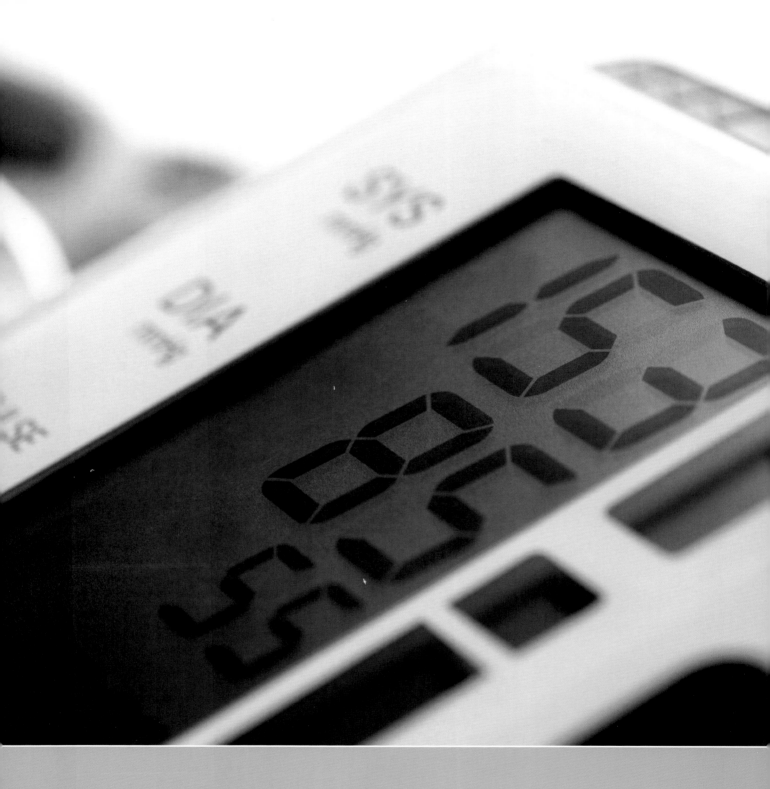

understanding & testing your body's health

At the start of any training programme, tests should be undertaken in order to monitor your progress and to demonstrate your eventual results. Ongoing testing also acts as a morale booster and highlights areas in which we are not performing to the best of our abilities. In this section we will look at why we are taking each test and then compare them to the recommendations from the governing bodies.

I opted for home testing throughout my 12-week programme instead of visiting my GP every week for the sake of convenience. Remember though, these tests are not as accurate as those you may receive from your doctor, so perhaps visit your GP before and after your 12-week plan, as I did. This will ensure both sets of your results are accurate and, if you do have any health concerns, your doctor will be able to diagnose and treat you.

Most of the home health testing kits are easily available on the high street from Boots, the UK's leading pharmacy, health and beauty retailer.

Equipment needed for the health tests

- Accurate scales
- Tape measure
- Boots glucose home test (One Touch Ultra2 Blood Glucose monitoring system)
- Boots cholesterol home test
- Callipers (purchased from internet)
- Body fat percentage reader (purchased from internet)
- Peak flow meter (purchased from internet)
- Watch
- Boots blood pressure monitor (Intellisense Blood Pressure Arm Monitor)

Height

This will give you no relevant information on its own, apart from telling you how tall or, in my case, how short you are! But this is a result you will need in order to work out your BMI test (Body Mass Index).

The tests

Every Week	Every 4 Weeks
Health tests	**Health tests**
Weight	All 7 weekly health tests.
Height	Postural test
BMI	Calliper test
Body Fat % test	Cholesterol
Blood pressure	Glucose
Resting heart rate	Lung function
Measurements	**Fitness tests**
	1 rep max – 4 exercises
	Max in 1 minute – 4 exercises
	Max pull ups

Full explanations on all of the fitness tests are available in the **Train to Become Fitness book**.

Weight / Scales

Jumping on the scales every day is not the most accurate way to follow your progress. It is a good guide but try not to put too much pressure on yourself to lose a specific amount of weight each week. Please note that I never weighed myself everyday as this can be very disheartening, so I would do it every Sunday on test day.

You will need to weigh yourself to work out your BMI, unless you do as I did with my results and use the fat percentage reader which automatically shows you the readings.

Body Mass Index (BMI)

There is no average weight or size that a person should be, but there is a method to discover if we fit into the general health practitioners' recommendations. Using height and weight measurements we can use the Body Mass Index (BMI) to determine a healthy weight for your height.

Using the BMI equation is a great and quick technique to work out which weight range that you are in, take note however that this should not be used by bodybuilders or athletes as they have a higher than normal amount of muscle mass.

The equation
Weight (kg) ÷ height (m) = then ÷ height (m) = BMI

For example if you weigh 80kg and you are 1.75m tall, your BMI would be 26.1 (80÷1.75= 45.7 then 45.7÷1.75=26.1). Using the chart below, you can see that the end figure would mean that the person is overweight.

For my BMI results I used a body fat percentage monitor for its calculations.

The BMI chart

Under weight	13–18
Normal weight	19–24
Overweight	25–29
Obese / Seriously overweight	30–40
Dangerously overweight / Morbidly obese	40 +

Blood Pressure (BP)

Checking blood pressure is essential as it directly affects your health. Blood pressure testing measures your heart beat and the strength of the oxygen pushing blood around the vessels in your body. An ideal, healthy blood pressure is 120 over 80. The first number is your systolic blood pressure – the highest pressure when your heart beats, and the second number is your diastolic blood pressure – the lowest pressure when your heart relaxes between beats.

The chart below shows the ideal in blood pressure types

	Systolic	Diastolic
Low	70 over 90	40 over 60
Ideal	90 over 120	60 over 80
Pre high	120 over 140	80 over 90
High	140 over 190 +	90 over 100+

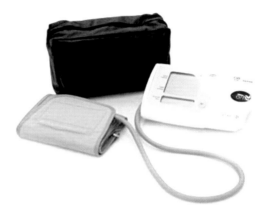

This is the blood pressure monitor that I used, the Boots Intellisense Blood Pressure Arm Monitor.

My blood pressure was at 130/92 in week 1 and after completing the 12-week challenge, was 127/44.

Resting Heart Rate (RHR)

This test measures your heart's efficiency in pumping blood around the body when you are in a resting state. The RHR is able to tell you how fit you are and by following the **Train to Become Fitness book** you should see a steady decrease in your heart rate as your heart becomes more efficient.

During the 12-week fitness and nutrition plan, I took my resting heart rate readings as soon as I woke up in the morning, to get my best record.

You can find your RHR by simply finding your pulse on the thumb side of the wrist and counting your heart beat for one minute with your index and middle finger to see what result you have.

At the beginning of week 1 my resting heart rate was 79 beats per minute and by the end of week 12 it had decreased to 37 beats per minute. The female's resting heart rate at the beginning of her fitness plan was 77 beats per minute and by the end of the fitness plan it had decreased to 50 beats per minute.

The table below shows the average RHR. Mark where you are on the table to see how fit you are right now and then mark it again in 12 weeks time?

Men						
Age	18–25	26–35	36–45	46–55	56–65	65+
Athlete	49–55	49–54	50–56	50–57	51–56	50–55
Excellent	56–61	55–61	57–62	58–63	57–61	56–61
Good	62–65	62–65	63–66	64–67	62–67	62–65
Above average	66–69	66–70	67–70	68–71	68–71	66–69
Average	70–73	71–74	71–75	72–76	72–75	70–73
Below average	74–81	75–81	76–82	77–83	76–81	74–79
Poor	82+	82+	83+	84+	82+	80+

Women						
Age	18–25	26–35	36–45	46–55	56–65	65+
Athlete	54–60	54–59	54–59	54–60	54–59	54–59
Excellent	61–65	60–64	60–64	61–65	60–64	60–64
Good	66–69	65–68	65–69	66–69	65–68	65–68
Above average	70–73	69–72	70–73	70–73	69–73	69–72
Average	74–78	73–76	74–78	74–77	74–77	73–76
Below average	79–84	77–82	79–84	78–83	78–83	77–84
Poor	85+	83+	85+	84+	84+	84+

Calliper Test

This test measures skin folds to calculate your body's fat percentage. You will need to have another person available to help take the measurements for this test, but again this can be done at home.

To take the calliper test:

- Use the left hand side for all of your measurements with your arms hanging freely.

- Pinch 1cm above the area being measured with the calliper.

- Measure all your calliper positions so that the next reading will be taken in the same place.

- The pinch should be maintained throughout the reading for a specific area before moving on towards the next area.

- Take the measurement a couple of times to gain the most accurate reading allowing the skin to return to normal between readings.

Areas to measure

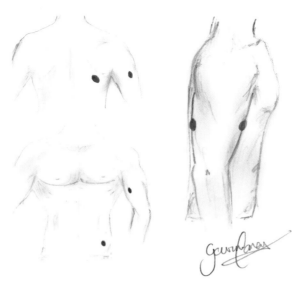

1. Biceps
Vertical fold for the pinch. Measure half way between the shoulder and the elbow directly onto the bicep to take the reading.

2. Triceps
Vertical fold for the pinch. Measure half way between the shoulder and the elbow directly onto the tricep to take the reading.

3. Suprailiac
Diagonal fold for the pinch. Measure directly above the hip.

4. Subscapular
Diagonal fold for the pinch. Measure 1-2cm down at 45° directly from the bottom of the shoulder blade.

Now add all four of your calliper measurements (biceps, triceps, superiliac and subscapular) together to get your total skin folds measurement.

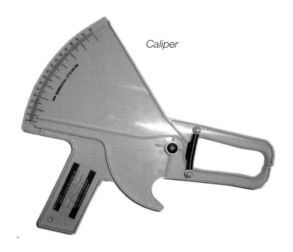

Caliper

Apply your total skin folds measurement to the appropriate tables below:

Average Male Calliper Test Results:

Total measurements for all four skin folds (mm)	Age 16–29 Fat %	Age 30–49 Fat %	Age 50 Fat %
Lean	**<8**	**<8**	**<8**
Optimal	8-15	11-17	12-19
Slightly overweight	**16-20**	**16-20**	**16-20**
Fat	21-24	21-24	21-24
Obese	**>25**	**>25**	**>25**
20	8.1	12.1	12.5
22	9.2	13.2	13.9
24	10.2	14.2	15.1
26	11.2	15.2	16.3
28	12.1	16.1	17.4
30	12.9	16.9	17.5
35	14.7	18.7	20.8
40	16.3	20.3	22.8
45	17.7	21.8	24.7
50	19.0	23.0	26.3
55	20.2	24.2	27.8
60	21.2	25.3	29.1
65	22.2	26.2	30.4
70	23.2	27.1	31.5
75	24.0	28.0	32.6
80	24.8	28.8	33.7
85	25.6	29.6	34.6
90	26.3	30.3	35.5
95	27.0	31.0	36.5
100	27.6	31.7	37.3
110	28.8	32.9	38.8
120	29.9	34.0	40.2
130	31.0	35.0	41.5
140	31.9	36.0	42.8
150	32.8	36.8	43.9

Average Female Calliper Test Results:

Total measurements for all four skin folds (mm)	Age 16–29 Fat %	Age 30–49 Fat %	Age 50 Fat %
Lean	**<8**	**<8**	**<8**
Optimal	8-15	11-17	12-19
Slightly overweight	**16-20**	**16-20**	**16-20**
Fat	21-24	21-24	21-24
Obese	**>25**	**>25**	**>25**
14	9.4	14.1	17
16	11.2	15.7	18.6
18	12.7	17.1	20.1
20	14.1	18.4	21.4
22	15.4	19.5	22.6
24	16.5	20.6	23.7
26	17.6	21.5	24.8
28	18.6	22.4	25.7
30	19.5	23.3	26.6
35	24.6	25.2	28.6
40	23.4	26.8	30.3
45	25	28.3	31.9
50	26.5	29.6	33.2
55	27.8	30.8	34.6
60	29.1	31.9	35.7
65	30.2	32.9	36.7
70	31.2	33.9	37.7
75	32.2	34.7	38.6
80	33.1	35.6	39.5
85	34	36.3	40.4
90	34.8	37.1	41.1
95	35.6	37.8	41.9
100	36.3	38.5	42.6
120	39	40.8	45.1
130	40.2	41.9	46.2
140	41.3	42.9	47.3
150	42.3	43.8	48.2

Measurements

I use measurements constantly with clients as well as in my own training as it is a great way to show how the body is reacting to your exercise and nutrition.

With the results of your measurements and your fat percentage, you will accurately be able to see if you are losing body fat rather than just losing weight (which may well just be fluid).

To take measurements accurately, you will need someone else to take them for you so your body can relax in a standing position. All my measurements were taken while I was cold and relaxed and they were taken roughly at the same time every Sunday throughout the 12-week plan.

Please take careful note of exactly where you are taking your measurements from and ensure that you measure from exactly the same place every time, in order to keep your results as precise and effective as possible.

Neck

Measure down from where the ear lobe and jaw connect. The measurement will be down to the largest part of the neck. Take a note of the measurement, then measure around the neck for the result.

Chest

Place the tape measure around the upper torso, measuring from the nipples and keeping the tape in the same alignment all of the way around.

Upper arm

Look at the arm and mark out the largest circumference. Measure up from the lateral epicondyle of the humerus (or the bony bit on the outside of the elbow!). Take note of the measurement and then measure around the circumference for the result. Repeat for the opposite arm.

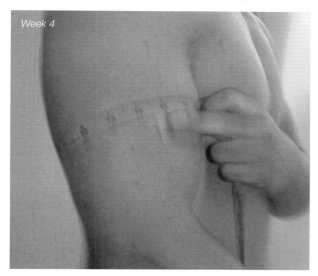

Week 4

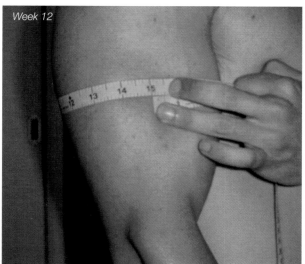

Week 12

Not bad in just 12 weeks, a gain of 1½ inches.

Waist/naval

Place the tape measure around your abdomen, measuring from the belly button and keeping the tape in alignment all the way around.

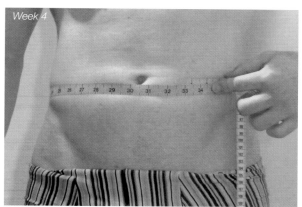

Week 4

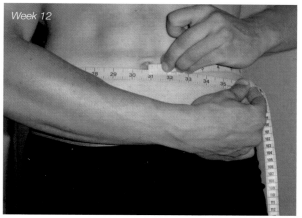

Week 12

I lost a lot of inches from my waist but this was not all body weight as you might think.

Hips

Place the tape measure around the hip over the anterior superior iliac spine (or the bony parts either side of your hip). Make sure the tape goes all of the way around and is in alignment with the front.

Upper thigh

Look at the widest part on the upper thigh and mark. Measure up from the head of the fibula (or the bony part on the outside of the top of the lower leg). Take note of the measurement and then measure around the circumference for the result and repeat for the opposite thigh.

Calf

Look at the largest part on the calf and measure around its circumference. Repeat for the opposite calf.

Body Fat Percentage Test

This is a quicker and more convenient version of the calliper test, however the results are not quite as accurate. I chose to do this test every week to allow me to see the change and keep me on track.

There are a number of body fat monitor models available and the model I purchased from the internet notes your BMI as well. I took a couple of readings from the monitor each time to make sure the readings were as accurate as possible. Most models are similar to normal bathroom scales which you stand on with bare feet. Other monitors, like mine, are handheld.

The monitor passes a low-level, imperceptible electric current through your body. As lean body tissue contains mainly water and electrolytes, this conducts the current throughout the body giving you a reading.

Fat, however, contains limited water and is not a good conductor, so it impedes the current. By measuring your lean body mass, the monitor can predict your fat mass.

For best results, the monitors should be used at the same time of day, once a week and wearing minimal clothing.

Note:
You need to empty your bladder before use, as this will affect the results. Also, avoid alcohol and use the device straight after exercising.

Have a look at the graph on page 38 to see the fantastic results we accomplished during the 12-week Train to Become Challenge (following all three books in the series).

Lung Function Test

Peak Expiratory Flow Rate (PEFR)
The lung function test is measured by a Peak Flow Meter, a small hand-held device used to measure how fast a person can exhale. This shows how well your airways are performing.

In the Female Fitness book, even though the female subject is an asthma sufferer you will see from her results later in the chapter, that her lung performance increases quite considerably due to improvements in her health and fitness levels.

To take the PEFR

1. Breathe in as deep as possible

2. Blow out into the meter as hard and as fast as possible

3. Take note of its result and repeat three times and record your highest rate.

See the graph of our results on page 38.

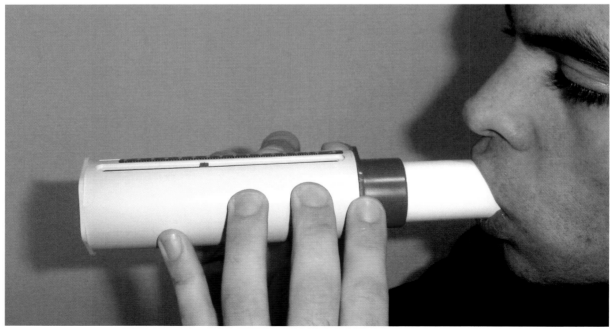

My lung function reading on the Peak Flow Meter increased from 600 to 700 as my fitness improved on the 12-week challenge.

MEN

AGE	Height 1.55m (5ft 1')	1.60m (5ft 3')	1.65m (5ft 5')	1.70m (5ft 7')	1.75m (5ft 9')	1.80m (5ft11')	1.85m (6ft 1')	1.90m (6ft 3')
25	515	534	552	570	589	607	625	644
30	502	520	539	557	576	594	612	632
35	489	508	526	544	563	582	600	619
40	476	495	513	531	550	568	586	606
45	463	482	501	519	537	556	574	593
50	450	469	487	505	524	543	561	580
55	438	456	475	493	511	530	548	567
60	424	443	462	480	498	517	535	545
65	412	430	449	460	486	504	522	541
70	399	417	436	545	472	491	509	528

WOMEN

AGE	Height: 1.45m (4ft 9')	1.50m (4ft11')	1.55m (5ft 1')	1.60m (5ft 3')	1.65m (5ft 5')	1.70m (5ft 7')	1.75m (5ft 9')	1.80m (5ft11')
25	365	383	400	416	433	449	466	482
30	357	374	390	407	423	440	456	473
35	348	365	381	398	414	431	447	464
40	339	356	372	389	405	422	438	455
45	330	347	363	380	397	413	429	446
50	321	338	354	371	388	404	420	437
55	312	329	345	362	379	395	411	428
60	303	320	336	353	370	386	402	419
65	294	311	327	344	361	377	393	410
70	285	302	318	335	352	368	384	401

Glucose Test

This test measures the amount of glucose in the blood and is used to detect hyperglycaemia (higher than normal glucose levels within the blood) and hypoglycaemia (lower than normal glucose levels within the blood). It also helps identify diabetes.

I chose to use the fasting blood glucose test for ease. This required me to eat no later than 10pm the night before and to take the test at around 8am the following morning. Keeping the test criteria the same provides the best results. Please read and follow the instructions carefully to the specific test kit that you use.

The result guidelines for the fasting blood glucose test I took are in the table below:

From 3.6 to 6.0 mmol/L	Normal fasting glucose
From 6.1 to 6.9 mmol/L	Impaired fasting glucose
7.0 mmol/L and above	Probable diabetes

Cholesterol Test

Our bodies need a certain amount of cholesterol to make cell membranes, insulate nerves and produce hormones. Cholesterol is a waxy substance produced in the liver and other organs. We can also absorb cholesterol from foods such as eggs, red meat, cheese and more. Too much or too high a cholesterol level can affect your heart.

There are two forms of cholesterol, one of which is good for you while the other is bad.

Good Cholesterol
High density lipoprotein (HDL) picks up and transports surplus cholesterol from the body tissues back to the liver where it is broken down and passed out of the body.

Bad Cholesterol
Low density lipoprotein (LDL) transports cholesterol from the liver around the rest of the body. When there is more LDL in the blood than the body needs, the cholesterol accumulates in the body tissues, such as the walls of the coronary arteries. Here that it can build up and affect the heart function.

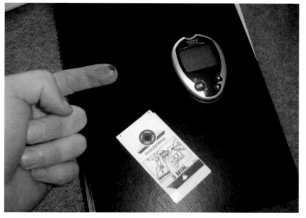

This cholesterol test gave me good readings but I never looked forward to pricking my finger every four weeks!

The home test kit that I used throughout the 12-week plan simply measured the total amount of cholesterol. Please remember to read and follow the instructions.

The levels of total cholesterol fall into the following categories:

Ideal level	3.9–5.2 mmol/l
Mildly high level	5.0–6.4 mmol/l
High level	6.5–7.8 mmol/l
Very high level	7.8+ mmol/l

Consider that muscle weighs more than fat, so sometimes while your weight may remain the same, your muscles are becoming stronger, more toned just like in my results. This is something to bear in mind when you look at your measurements and fat percentage readings.

Remember – this is not a guide as to how fit and healthy you are. Everybody is different and unique, these are simply our results over the 12 weeks to show you the amazing difference you can achieve if you're 100% committed as we were.

12 week plan – Our test results

The following statistics and measurements show all of the tests that we used and details explicitly how our bodies changed over the entire 12-week plan. You will see that we used a range of tests to observe how our bodies were reacting to the plan, from simple weight and height measurements to the calliper test used to assess body fat and the fitness test. Use these as an outline to help set up your own tests so that you can see how your body responds to the 12-week plan.

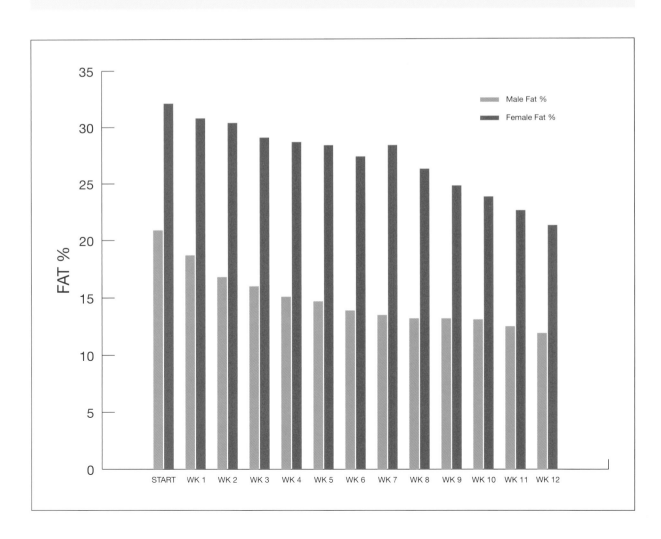

Male overall results – increases and decreases

Health Statistics

Weight (kg):	- 9.5
Height (cm):	175 ½

Measurements (inches):

Neck:	- 1
Chest:	+ 3
Arms:	R + 1 ½, L + 1 ¼ inches
Navel:	- 4 ¾
Hips:	- 2 ½
Thighs:	R + ½ inch, L + 1 inch
Calves:	R same, L + ½ inch

Calliper Test (mm):

Bicep:	- 4
Tricep:	- 2
Waist:	- 8
Subscapularis:	- 4
Total:	- 18
Calliper fat %:	- 6.9
Postural Test	See Postural Section, Chapter 5
Glucose:	- 1.0
Cholesterol:	- 2.0
BMI:	- 2.8
Fat %:	- 9
Blood Pressure:	- 6/48
Resting Heart Rate:	- 42
Lung Function:	+ 100

Fitness Tests

Bleep test (20 m) level: Gained over 2.5 levels

Maximum reps in 1 minute:

Push ups:	+ 29
½ sit ups:	+ 41
Squats:	+ 37
Dips:	+ 36
Maximum pull ups:	+ 30

1 rep maximum weight training (kg):

Squats:	+ 27.5
Bench Press:	+ 30
Military Press:	+ 12.5
Deadlifts: Gained	+ 20

Female Overall Results – Increases and Decreases

Health Statistics

Weight (kg):	- 4.5
Height (cm):	157.3

Measurements (inches)

Neck:	- 1
Chest:	- 2 ¾
Arms:	R – 1 ¼, L - 1
Navel:	- 4
Hips:	- 5
Thighs:	R – 2 ¾, L – 2 ¼
Calves:	R – ½, L – ½

Calliper Test

Bicep:	- 3
Tricep:	- 10
Waist:	- 8
Subscapularis:	- 9
Total:	- 30
Calliper fat %:	- 8.6
Postural Test	See Postural Section, Chapter 5
Glucose:	- 2.4
Cholesterol:	- 1.3
BMI:	- 1.8
Fat %:	- 10.8
Blood Pressure:	- 2/7
Resting Heart Rate:	- 27
Lung Function:	+ 80

Fitness Tests

Bleep test (20m) level: Gained over 3.5 levels

Max reps in 1 min

Push ups:	+ 30
½ sit ups:	+ 38
Squats:	+ 42
Dips:	+ 47
Maximum pull ups:	+ 4 ½

You will have your own results table to fill in every week, within the **Train to Become Fitness book** and then you can compare your results to the tables within this book.

Male results

Sunday 15 March 2009		
Statistics		
Weight (kg):		87.5
Height (cm):		175.5
Measurements (inches)		
Neck:	16	
Chest:	39	
Arms:	R 13 ½ L 13 ¾	
Navel:	35 ½	
Hips:	34 ½	
Thighs:	R 24 L 23 ½	
Calves:	R 16 L 15 ½	
Calliper Test (mm)		
Bicep:		6
Tricep:		8
Waist:		15
Subscapularis:		12
Total:		41
Calliper fat %:		16.6
BMI:		28.1
Fat %:		20.9
BP:		133 / 92
RHR:		79
Glucose:		5.9
Cholesterol:		5.9
Lung Function:		600
Fitness Tests		
Bleep test (level): 10.7		
Maximum reps in one minute		
Push ups:		59
½ sit ups:		60
Squats:		52
Dips:		55
Max pull ups:		12
1 rep maximum weight training (kg)		
Squats:		110
Bench Press:		100
Military Press:		60
Deadlifts:		120

Sunday 12 April 2009		
Statistics		
Weight (kg):		80
Height (cm):		175 ½
Measurements (inches)		
Neck:	15 ¼	
Chest:	41	
Arms:	R 14 ½ L 14 ½	
Navel:	32 ¾	
Hips:	34	
Thighs:	R 24 L 24	
Calves:	R 15 ¾ L 15¾	
Calliper Test (mm)		
Bicep:		3
Tricep:		7
Waist:		10
Subscapularis:		11
Total:		31
Calliper fat %:		13.1
BMI:		26.0
Fat %:		15.1
BP:		140 / 58
RHR:		57
Glucose:		5.7
Cholesterol:		4.6
Lung Function:		640
Fitness Tests		
Bleep test (level): 12.3		
Maximum reps in one minute		
Push ups:		74
½ sit ups:		91
Squats:		72
Dips:		80
Max pull ups:		27
1 rep maximum weight training (kg)		
Squats:		120
Bench Press:		110
Military Press:		62 ½
Deadlifts:		125

Sunday 10 May 2009		
Statistics		
Weight (kg):		78.5
Height (cm):		175 ½
Measurements (inches)		
Neck:	15 ¼	
Chest:	41 ¾	
Arms:	R 14 ¾ L 14 ¾	
Navel:	31 ¼	
Hips:	32 ¾	
Thighs:	R 24 ¼ L 24 ¼	
Calves:	R15 ¾ L15 ¾	
Calliper Test (mm)		
Bicep:		3
Tricep:		6
Waist:		9
Subscapularis:		9
Total:		27
Calliper fat %:		11.9
BMI:		25.5
Fat %:		13.2
BP:		138 / 44
RHR:		45
Glucose:		5.1
Cholesterol:		3.9
Lung Function:		670
Fitness Tests		
Bleep test (level): 12.5		
Maximum reps in one minute		
Push ups:		80
½ sit ups:		99
Squats:		78
Dips:		90
Max Pull ups:		35
1 rep maximum weight training (kg)		
Squats:		132 ½
Bench Press:		120
Military Press:		64
Deadlifts:		132 ½

Sunday 7 June 2009		
Statistics		
Weight (kg):		78
Height (cm):		175 ½
Measurements (inches)		
Neck:	15	
Chest:	42	
Arms:	R 15 L 15	
Navel:	30 ¾	
Hips:	32	
Thighs:	R 24 ½ L 24 ½	
Calves:	R 16 L 16	
Calliper Test (mm)		
Bicep:		2
Tricep:		6
Waist:		7
Subscapularis:		8
Total:		23
Calliper fat %:		9.7
BMI:		25.3
Fat %:		11.9
BP:		127 / 44
RHR:		37
Glucose:		4.9
Cholesterol:		3.9
Lung Function:		700
Fitness Tests		
Bleep test (level): 13.4		
Maximum reps in one minute		
Push ups:		88
½ sit ups:		101
Squats:		89
Dips:		91
Max Pull ups:		42
1 rep maximum weight training (kg)		
Squats:		137 ½
Bench Press:		130
Military Press:		72 ½
Deadlifts:		140

Ready to lose the weight now. I didn't like the way I looked or felt.

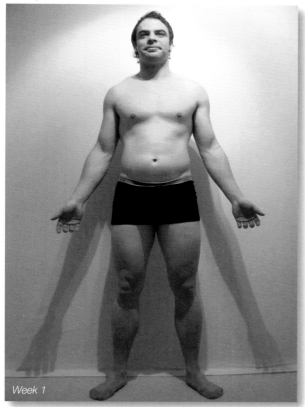

Week 1

At this early stage you can notice me starting to lose weight.

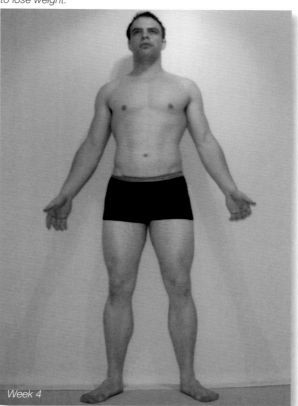

Week 4

I am now starting to take shape and my physique is becoming more muscular.

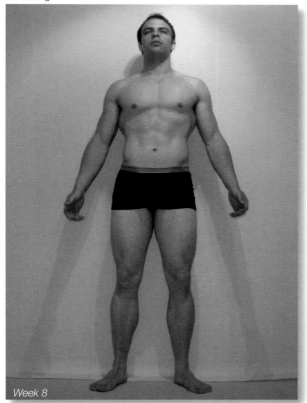

Week 8

By week 12, I was so happy that I had reached my ultimate goal. I hope you can get the body you want too!

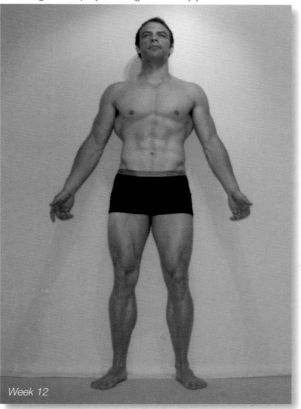

Week 12

Female results

Sunday 5 July 2009		Sunday 2 August 2009		Sunday 30 August 2009		Sunday 27 September 2009	
Statistics		**Statistics**		**Statistics**		**Statistics**	
Weight (kg):	57	Weight (kg):	55	Weight (kg)	53 ½	Weight (kg):	52 ½
Height (cm):	157.3	Height (cm):	157.3	Height (cm) :	157.3	Height (cm):	157.3
Measurements (inches)		**Measurements (inches)**		**Measurements (inches)**		**Measurements (inches)**	
Neck:	12 ¼	Neck:	12	Neck:	11 ¾	Neck:	11 ¼
Chest:	35 ½	Chest:	33 ¼	Chest:	32 ¾	Chest:	32 ¾
Arms:	R 11 ¾ L 11 ½	Arms:	R 11 L 11	Arms:	R 10 ¾ L 10 ¾	Arms:	R 10 ½ L 10 ½
Navel:	32'	Navel:	30 ¼	Navel:	29 ¼	Navel:	28
Hips:	36	Hips:	33	Hips:	31 ½	Hips:	31
Thighs:	R 23 ¾ L 23 ¼	Thighs:	R 22 ¾ L 22 ¾	Thighs:	R 22 L 22	Thighs:	R 21 L 21
Calves:	R 14 L 14	Calves:	R 14 L 14	Calves:	R 14 L 14	Calves:	R 13 ½ L 13 ½
Calliper test (mm)		**Calliper test (mm)**		**Calliper test (mm)**		**Calliper test (mm)**	
Bicep:	8	Bicep:	8	Bicep:	6	Bicep:	5
Tricep:	18	Tricep:	16	Tricep:	12	Tricep:	8
Waist:	15	Waist:	11	Waist:	8	Waist:	7
Subscapularis:	19	Subscapularis:	15	Subscapularis:	12	Subscapularis:	10
Total:	60	Total:	50	Total:	38	Total:	30
Calliper fat %:	31.9	Calliper fat %:	29.6	Calliper fat %:	26.1	Calliper fat %:	23.3
BMI:	23	BMI:	22.2	BMI:	21.6	BMI:	21.2
Fat %:	32.1	Fat %:	28.7	Fat %:	26.3	Fat %:	21.3
BP:	112 / 68	BP:	123 / 67	BP:	110 / 66	BP:	110 / 61
RHR:	77	RHR:	59	RHR:	58	RHR:	50
Glucose:	6.2	Glucose:	5.3	Glucose:	3.8	Glucose:	3.8
Cholesterol:	5.2	Cholesterol:	4.6	Cholesterol:	3.9	Cholesterol:	3.9
Lung function:	370	Lung function:	390	Lung function:	420	Lung function:	450
Fitness tests		**Fitness tests**		**Fitness tests**		**Fitness tests**	
Bleep test (20m) level: 4.5		Bleep test (20m) level: 5		Bleep test (20m) level: 6.7		Bleep test (20m) level: 8	
Maximum reps in one minute		**Maximum reps in one minute**		**Maximum reps in one minute**		**Maximum reps in one minute**	
Push ups ¾ :	15	Push ups ¾:	24	Push ups ¾:	35	Push ups ¾:	45
½ sit ups:	35	½ sit ups:	42	½ sit ups:	60	½ sit ups:	73
Squats:	39	Squats:	43	Squats:	59	Squats:	81
Dips:	23	Dips:	30	Dips:	51	Dips:	70
Max pull ups:	½	Max pull ups:	1	Max pull ups:	2 ½	Max pull ups:	5

The female was not that happy with herself when she started the 12 week plan!

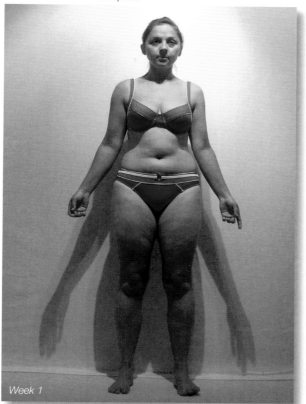

Week 1

What a difference already

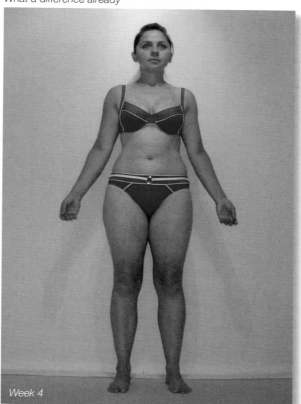

Week 4

You can really see the toning up, especially in the stomach area

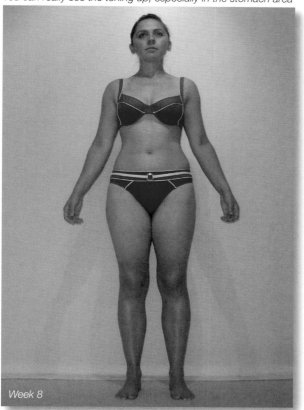

Week 8

The photo and results speak for themselves

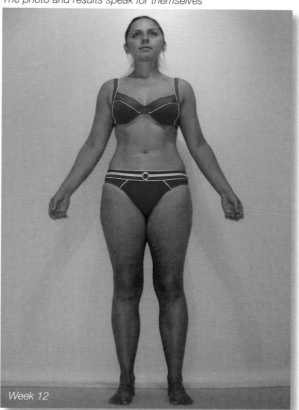

Week 12

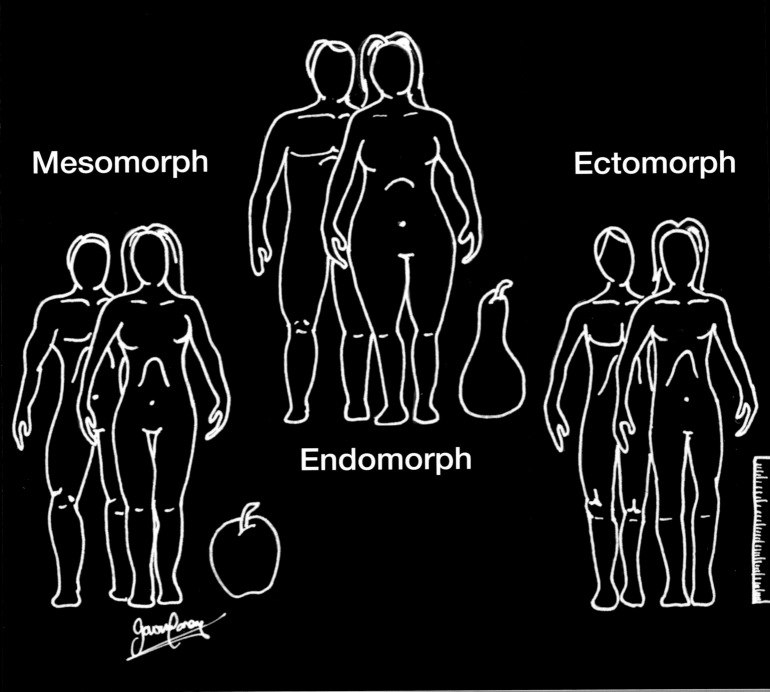

Mesomorph

Ectomorph

Endomorph

know your body type & posture

Our bodies come in many different shapes and sizes; some are short while others are tall, some are naturally slimmer, while others are larger. To achieve the correct posture as well as have a leaner, more toned and better proportioned body, you must first know which body type (Somatotype) you are and what kind of posture you have.

Recognising your body type

There is a popular method called 'Somatotype' which categorises the three main body types that we have: Ectomorph, Mesomorph and Endomorph. This does not mean however that you fit into just one category – most of us fall into two of these categories with different ratios.

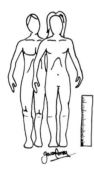

Ectomorph

Body type
Commonly known as the ruler and is characterised by a short upper body, long arms, legs and extremities.

This type has a small level of fat, but what they do have tends to occur around the middle. They have narrowness in the chest and shoulders with a tendency of an even smaller lower body with long thin muscles.

Foods to watch out for
This type craves simple carbohydrates like bread, cakes and biscuits and has a sweet tooth.

Notes for Ectomorphs
You tend to put on excess fat on the stomach and are the most likely to get Type 2 diabetes out of all the body types. You can also be overeaters and run a risk of heart disease and higher cholesterol than any of the other body types.

The right diet is essential to regulate this body type correctly, as weight is lost easily with the correct diet.

Exercise training for Ectomorphs
As you are leaner than the other body types you are best to build muscle with power movement so learn to train yourself hard but remember to give yourself plenty of rest and water.

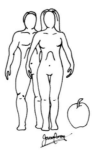

Mesomorph

Body type
Otherwise known as the apple shape and is characterised by shoulders and hips which tend to be the same width, a large chest, large torso, solid muscle structure with long legs and is well proportioned.

Foods to watch out for
This body type is able to eat most foods without being too concerned.

Notes for Mesomorphs
You lose weight more easily than the other body types and tend to build muscle easily and your risk of cardiovascular disease is less.

Exercise training for Mesomorphs
You will have to change your exercise routine regularly as your body type becomes used to a routine quickly.

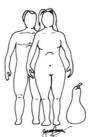

Endomorph

Body type
Known as the pear shape and is characterised by wide hips and thighs and are bottom heavy, which does actually make your legs appear smaller. This body type has a tendency to look flat or droopy and is the largest of the body types.

Foods to watch out for
This type tends to crave dairy and high fat foods.

Notes for Endomorphs
You run a lower risk for cardiovascular disease than Ectomorphs and normally gain weight around the hips. You will find it harder than the other body types to lose weight and a good diet is needed so as to not put on too much weight.

Training for Endomorphs
As you tend to be the larger body type your body will work best with high repetition training like cardiovascular and aerobic exercise such as running and swimming.

Posture

Posture plays such an important role in the health of your body, but more often than not is simply overlooked. The ideal skeletal alignment and consequent good posture involves teaching your body to stand, lie, walk and sit in positions that require the least amount of strain on supporting ligaments during any body movement. Having good posture keeps bones and joints in the correct alignment so muscles are used correctly. It prevents fatigue because muscles are being used more effectively and therefore using less energy and even contributes to a good appearance – more supermodel, less hunchback!

The easiest way to see if you have a good posture is to stand next to a plumb line, this represents gravity, to see if any body parts are out of sink. I use this method with clients and on myself to identify any postural faults and to help to distinguish which areas I need to strengthen or release. Please note, you will need someone to help you with this test.

At the back of this book is the **Myo Stretch Routine**, use this to guide you into using the correct stretches and use the **Train to Become Fitness book** for the correct exercises.

The set up

Postural alignment equipment

- White, clear wall to stand in front of
- Picture hook to hang plumb line from
- Coloured string to reach from the ceiling to 2cm above the floor.
- Plumb bob available from any DIY store
- Tape measure to measure feet position
- Camera to take images of your posture

Procedure and setup of the plumb line test

1. Tie one end of the coloured string to the plumb bob.
2. With the other end, tie in a loop to hang onto the picture hook from the ceiling.

Remember, this method is not as accurate as if you were to visit a health professional but it is something that can be done at home.

Front view

Use the instructions below to take photos of your posture for the front view.

1. Stand bare foot with your feet hip width apart either side of the plumb line and ask someone to measure the distance from the plumb line to the inside base of your big toe. Do the same for the other foot.

2. Next, measure the gap between your feet from the base of both big toes. You now know where to position yourself next time, quickly and easily.

3. While standing in this position, in front of a white, clear wall take around five photographs to analyse your posture with reference to the plumb line.

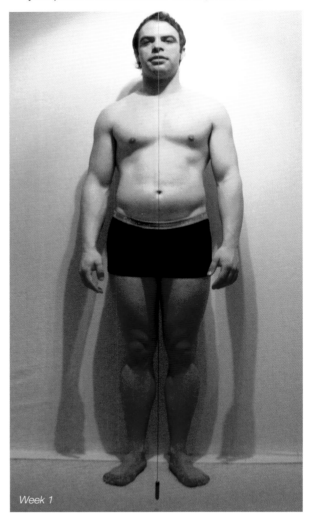

Week 1

This front view from week 1 shows you how far apart your feet should be. Also notice my white stomach!

Side view

The side view posture test hypothetically divides the body into front and back sections of equal weight. To examine your side view posture, follow these instructions.

1. Stand bare foot, side on to the plumb line.

2. Ask someone to position you correctly so the plumb line passes slightly forward to the ankle and approximately through the apex of the arch. In this position, measure from the heel to the wall and repeat for the other foot.

3. Apply the same measurement for the gap between your feet in the same manner as above.

4. Standing in your position in front of a white, clear wall take around five photographs to analyse your posture.

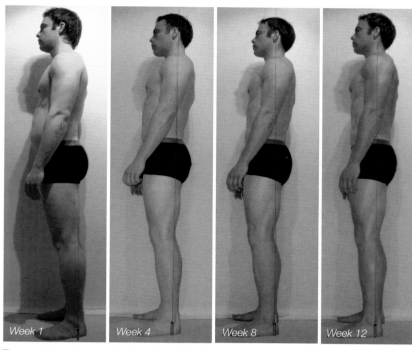

Week 1   Week 4   Week 8   Week 12

These photos show you the transformation that your body will undergo through 12 weeks. It is amazing how with the right training, stretching, and nutrition routines and with a little help from the Myo massage, your posture can be corrected.

Analysing your posture

Your posture provides a lot of information about the state of your body. Postural analysis allows you to see which areas of the body are under more stress than others, which could result in back ache, which I was experiencing before starting the 12-week health, fitness and nutrition books.

Analyse, compare and diagnose your own posture to that of a neutral posture using the following guidelines and pictures. If you have a misaligned posture then use the relevant information given to strengthen or stretch your muscles to realign yourself.

Again the results speak for themselves, but you may also notice the weight loss as well. This plays just as an important role as everything else mentioned.

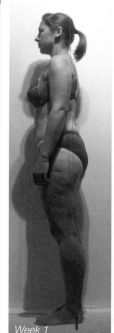 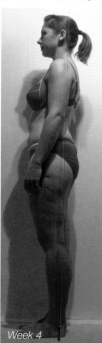 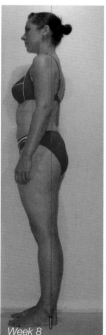 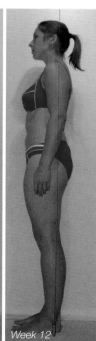

Week 1   Week 4   Week 8   Week 12

- Strong Muscles

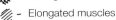 - Elongated muscles

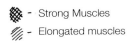

Neutral posture

The plumb line should pass through the following areas:

Head
Side view: lobe of the ear
Front view: centre of the head

Cervical spine
Side view: the neck represents a normal anterior curve
Front view: centre of the neck

Thoracic
Side view: the thoracic spine should curve slightly in a posterior direction and the plumb line should pass midway through the shoulder joint
Front view: centre of the chest

Lumbar
Side view: the lumbar should curve slightly anterior
Front view: centre and the naval

Pelvis
Side view: the front (anterior) and the back (posterior) of your hip should be at the same angle.

Hip joint
Side view: slightly posterior to the centre of the hip.
Front view: centre of your hips

Knee
Side view: slightly anterior through the axis of the knee joint. The knee should be neither flexed nor extended
Front view: directly in between your thighs and knees and with the same distance either side of the plumb line

Ankle
Side view: pass the ankle and through the apex of the arch of the foot
Front view: directly in between your calves and ankles and with the same distance either side of the plumb line

Feet
Your feet should be in a neutral position, with your toes angled outward slightly approximately 8 to 10 degrees and your heels together.

*To find out whether you have flat or pronated feet, look at the **Train to Become Fitness book**. This will help you identify in detail which gait (foot type) you have.*

Strengthen & Stretch

There are no elongated, weak, short and strong muscles. All the muscles are working in harmony with each other.

Kyphotic posture

Rounded and elongated upper back, the following describes the kyphotic posture from a side view.

Head	Forward
Cervical spine	Hyper extended (curves anteriorly more than normal)
Thoracic	Increased flexion (increased posterior curve / rounded shoulders)
Lumbar	Neutral
Pelvis	Neutral
Hip joint	Flexed
Knee	Normal / Neutral
Ankle	Normal / Neutral

Strengthen

Elongated or weak muscles
Neck flexors, upper back, external obliques, and hamstrings (slightly elongated but may or may not be weak). To aid your posture you need to exercise these muscles.

Exercises to help
These are just a few exercises to help realign your posture, which you can find in the **Train to Become Fitness book:**

- Reverse shrugs
- Bent over lat raises
- T-Bar Row

Stretch

Short or strong muscles.
The neck extensors and possibly your pectorals.

Stretches to help
Look at the Myo Stretch routine to find:

- Static stretch for the chest on a wall trapezius stretch
- Static stretch for the trapezius muscles

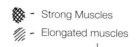

⬣ - Strong Muscles

⬳ - Elongated muscles

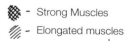

⬣ - Strong Muscles

⬳ - Elongated muscles

Lordotic posture

Means having a bigger arch in the lower back, the following describes the lordotic posture from a side view.

Head	Neutral
Cervical spine	Normal / Neutral (slight anterior)
Thoracic	Normal / Neutral (slight posterior)
Lumbar	Hyper-extended (a greater curve in your lower back)
Pelvis	Anterior tilt (the pelvis tilts forwards down more than normal)
Hip joint	Flexed
Knee	Slightly hyper-extended (knee is extended more than normal)
Ankle	Slight plantar flexion (your toes will point down towards the floor more than normal. This relates to you leaning on your toes)

Strengthen

Elongated or weak muscles

Abdominals and hamstrings may or may not be elongated. To help your posture you need to exercise these muscles.

Exercises to help

These are just a few exercises to help realign your posture, which you can find in the **Train to Become Fitness book:**

* Reverse curl
* Reverse crunch
* Stiff leg deadlifts

Stretch

Short or strong muscles

Lower back and hip flexor / rectus femoris. To help your posture you need to stretch these muscles.

Stretches to help

Look at the **Myo Stretch routine** to find:

* PNF Stretch for quad lying face down
* Developmental stretch for the lower back whilst lying down
* Developmental stretch for hip flexor stretch

Flat back

No or limited arch in the lower back, the following describes the flat back posture from a side view.

Head	Forward
Cervical spine	Slightly extended (causing your head to tilt up)
Thoracic	Increased flexion at the top and towards the bottom it straightens up. (Round shoulders into a straight lower back)
Lumbar	Hyper-flexed (the lower back becomes straight)
Pelvis	Posterior tilt (the pelvis tilts backwards / up more than normal)
Hip Jjoint	Extended
Knee	Slightly hyper-extended (knee is extended more than normal)
Ankle	Normal /Neutral

Strengthen

Elongated or weak muscles

Hip flexors and the back may seem elongated with a flat back but they may not be weak. To help your posture you need to exercise these muscles.

Exercises to help

These are just a few exercises to help realign your posture, which you can find in the **Train to Become Fitness book:**

* Reverse crunch
* Deadlifts
* Dorsal raises

Stretch

Short or strong muscles

Hamstrings and the abdominals are frequently strong. To help your posture you need to stretch these muscles.

Stretches to help

Look at the **Myo Stretch routine** to find:

* PNF stretch for hamstring muscles
* Developmental stretch for sitting hamstring muscles
* Static stretch for the abdominal muscles

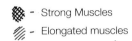

\- Strong Muscles
\- Elongated muscles

Sway back posture

The pelvis sways forward over the feet, causesing the hip joint to extend. The pelvis tilt makes the lumber spine flatten. This causes a long curve from the upper back to the lower back. The following describes the sway back posture from a side view.

Head	Forward
Cervical spine	Slightly extended (causing your head to tilt up)
Thoracic	Increased flexion (long kyphosis)
Lumbar	Flexion (flattening of the lower back)
Pelvis	Posterior tilt (the pelvis tilts backwards / up more than normal)
Hip joint	Hyper-extended
Knee	Slightly hyper-extended (knee is extended more than normal)
Ankle	Slight plantar flexion (your toes will point down towards the floor more than normal. This relates to you leaning on your toes.

Strengthen

Elongated or weak muscles

Hip joint flexors, external oblique, upper back extensors and neck extensors. To help your posture you need to exercise these muscles.

Exercises to help

These are just a few exercises to help realign your posture, which you can find in the **Train to Become Fitness book:**

- Bent over row
- Single arm cable row

Stretch

Short or strong muscles

Hamstrings and the upper part of the internal oblique. Lower back is normally strong but not short. To help your posture you need to stretch these muscles.

Front view – with the front views you should look for deviations where your pelvis, spine and shoulders are tilting slightly towards one side.

Stretches to help

Look at the **Myo Stretch routine** to find:

- Developmental stretch for sitting hamstring muscles
- PNF stretch for hamstring muscles

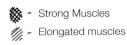

\- Strong Muscles
\- Elongated muscles

C shape posture

An ordinary C shape posture is when the shoulder is lower on the same side as the raised hip. The following describes the c shape posture from a side view.

Head	Normal / Neutral
Cervical spine	Normal / Neutral
Shoulder	Look to see if the shoulders are elevated, adducted, or slightly depressed. (This means the shoulder may be raised up, in or down).
Thoracic	Slight curvature either towards the left or right.
Lumbar	Slight curvature either towards the left or right.
Pelvis	Lateral tilt on the left or right(higher on one side than the other).
Hip joint	Adducted and slightly medial rotated on one side and abducted on the other side (one side is brought slightly forward and in / down and the other is higher.
Knee	Normal/Neutral
Ankle	Slight pronated (your feet may be rolled inwards, like flat feet)

Strengthen

Elongated or weak muscles

The side of your curvature depends on your muscles' strengths and weaknesses. The side where the pelvis is tilted lower is the weak side, so look at the weakness on the lateral trunk muscles, the hip adductors (inside thigh), inside of the left calf muscles and on the opposite side the hip abductors (gluteus medius muscle), and also look at the TFL (front of hip weakness). To help aid your posture you need to exercise these muscles.

Stretch

Short or strong muscles

Hamstrings and the abdominals are frequently strong. Using the same example, finding out the short or strong muscles is simple – it is the opposite of the weak muscles. For instance, the hip/pelvis that is raised/tilted up has tight lateral muscles, hip adductors (inside thigh), inside calf muscles and on the opposite side the abductors (Gluteus Medius muscle) and also look at the TFL (front of hip). To help aid your posture you need to stretch these muscles.

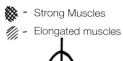

- Strong Muscles
- Elongated muscles

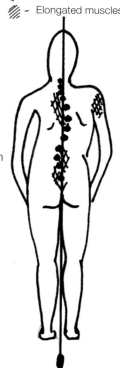

Scoliosis

The best way to diagnose Scoliosis is to have an examination in which the professional observes the movement in your back. An ordinary S-shape posture is when the shoulder is higher on the same side as the raised hip.

There are many reasons why you may suffer from scoliosis including.

- Injury
- Disease
- Changes in bone structure
- Shortness in one leg
- Impairment in hearing or vision
- Neuromuscular problems

Help to realign your posture

Now you can identify which category your posture falls into, you can take the correct steps to amend it by strengthening and shortening the weak muscles with exercise and by elongating the short but strong muscles by stretching them.

There are numerous exercises to realign your posture that can be found in the *Train to Become Fitness book.* There are many ways to help alleviate muscular tension that includes massage and stretching, both of which I've used to release tense muscles of my own.

Your Notes

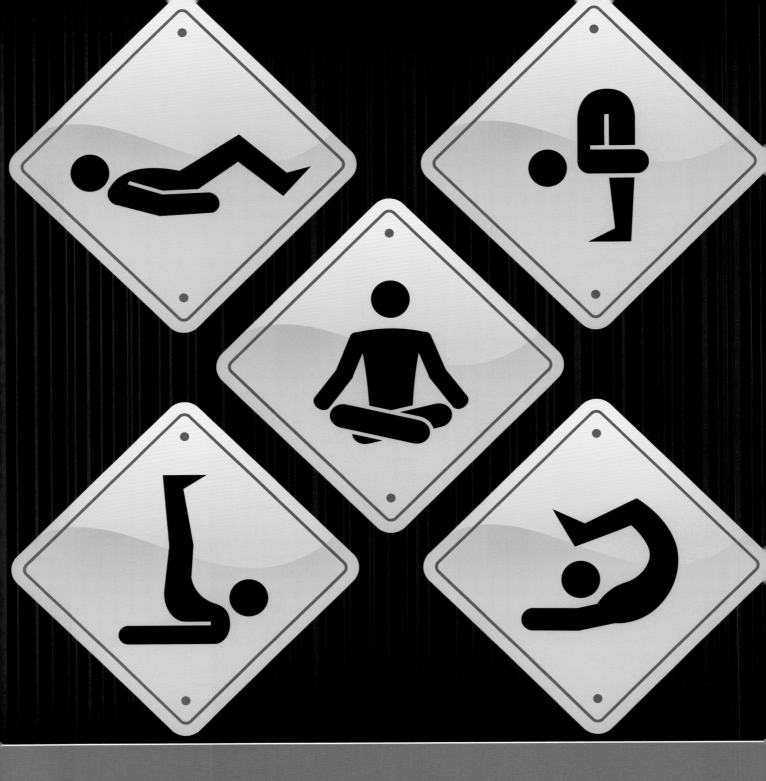

release the pressure

Massage is one of the oldest and simplest forms of medical care used to ease pain, anxiety and to promote good health. Massage therapy and stretching provides relaxation and relief to muscle strain and fatigue and this contributes to our overall health and wellbeing.

Massage

Massage therapy provides relaxation for both our mind and body. The results you get depend on the sort of massage you are going to receive.

I have chosen massages that help relieve muscular spasms and tension, aid in the breaking down of cellulite, boost the immune system and stimulate the lymphatic system.

The benefits of massage therapy are almost endless and include physical, emotional and physiological improvements to the body.

I used the Myo Clinic and Lush Spa for all the massages mentioned in these **Train to Become books**.

Myo Clinic

The Myo Clinic was founded by myself and simply means The Muscle Clinic. It was established with the philosophy that for the ultimate in health and wellbeing, you need a balance of health, fitness and nutrition. I believe in this idea so much that I've written three books about each. The book about health is what you are reading now!

The Myo Clinic employs different massages to achieve different results from within the body. We offer a range of unique programmes from weight loss to medical care. We use our extensive skills and knowledge in the human anatomy, along with the natural powers of pure essential oils, to achieve great results that anyone can be proud of.

Doctors, health practitioners publications such as GQ magazine have recognised the Myo Clinic for its unique and effective massages. The magazine GQ refered to the Myo Massage Method as a 'unique muscle release technique'.

Medical acupuncturist, Dr Clark, explains: 'Myo consultant Gavin treated me for persisting lower back/buttock pain using deep, manual massage with a unique pressure point therapy. He also instructed me on post-treatment exercises and a stretching regime'. Dr Clark goes on to say 'I am glad to say that Gavin's treatment helped resolve my condition. As a practicing medical acupuncturist I have no hesitation in recommending him to my own patients, friends and family'.

Below are some of the massages used during the 12 weeks. Not all of these massages aim to be relaxing but are all results based.

The Myo massage

Myo massage (the muscle massage)
This massage utilises specific techniques including a unique muscle release technique which I discovered during my travels abroad, even picking up tips from a witch doctor in the Solomon Islands! We also use pressure or trigger points and the very best of essential oils to work with massage to eliminate pain patterns. This approach ultimately brings balance between the musculoskeletal system and the nervous system.

Myo Lymphatic massage
This massage features special pumping strokes and vibrations to enhance the flow of the lymphatic system. Lymph is a whitish coloured liquid that flows throughout the body inside lymph vessels, which collect waste and toxins that cannot be absorbed through the capillary blood vessels. The combined movement and pressure encourages the movement of lymphatic fluid. This helps the immune and lymph systems, plus any other types of oedema, to return to full health and correct working order.

Myo Cellulite massage
This uses a distinctive technique that picks up and rolls the connective tissue, skin, fascia and adipose tissue (fat) to separate them from each other. It helps release the build up of cellulite which is then pushed to other specific areas with special strokes, to enable a fitness regime to take effect.

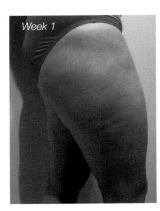 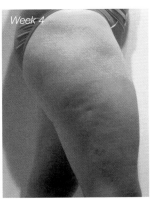 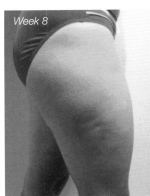 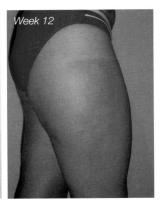

Week 1 *Week 4* *Week 8* *Week 12*

See the reduction in cellulite from following the **Train to Become Challenge** *and with a little help from the cellulite and lymphatic massages.*

The Myo Cellulite and the Myo Lymphatic Drainage massages were used on the female during her 12-week programme. This was done on a weekly basis and you can clearly see from the photos above the dramatic breakdown of cellulite and improvement in skin texture achieved during the 12-week programme.

The Myo massage techniques combined with the **Train to Become Fitness Plan**, the **Train to Become Nutrition Guide**, along with drinking plenty of water, completely changed the look of the skin around the thighs and on the stomach.

Lush Spa

I have to say, the Lush Spa is something very special. It has been in the making for decades and it is fantastic that now it is coming to flourition. Combining the scent of the English countryside, the comfort of a cosy English kitchen, the sound of beautiful birdsong and a nice, traditional cup of tea, Lush creates the ultimate and somewhat unique spa experience, based entirely as it is on Synaesthesia.

Synaesthesia is a unique therapy created by Lush founder Mark Constantine, hypnotherapist Lady Helen Kennedy, The Imagined Village's Simon Emerson and myself, Gavin Morey.

Synaesthesia Massage
This is the Lush signature spa treatment and is a combination of sensory stimulation designed to reinvent massage treatment and allow the client to drift into a receptive psychological state. With the choice of 11 different massage experiences, each one associated with different key words/phrases massage, they provide a sense of wellbeing. Using an individually prescribed

combination of scent (essential oils linked to a specific state of mind), sound (music especially composed for Lush where a birdsong is played), touch (with massage movements choreographed to music similar to that of classic ballet music), sight (with dry ice and colour therapy) and finally taste (includes a specially tailored tea) to complete your treatment experience.

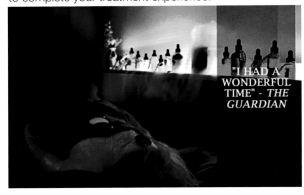

"I HAD A WONDERFUL TIME" - *THE GUARDIAN*

The new Lush Spa looks amazing….

With all of these elements working together in harmony, it allows you to relax enough to open your subconscious and help achieve the state of mind you originally chose from the choice of 11 key words at the beginning of your treatment journey, for example: confidence.

Myo Stretching by the Myo Clinic

Stretching is the process of placing a particular body part into a position that will lengthen the muscle and its associated soft tissue. As we stretch, other tissues like scar tissue, ligaments, tendons, fascia and skin also adapt. We stretch instinctively when we wake from sleep, have periods of inactivity or when leaving cramped spaces.

Throughout my 12-week fitness plan, I used the Myo Stretch, which is an hour-long stretching routine. The Myo Stretch encompasses and works the majority of the muscles within your body. Personally, I did this routine every Sunday and worked on those specific muscles which felt tight.

There are multiple benefits to stretching and it should not be overlooked in your daily health routine. When we stretch properly we:

- Increase our range of motion (ROM)
- Increase performance in training and exercise (power and strength)
- Improve posture
- Reduce fatigue within muscles
- Reduce any delayed onset of muscle soreness after training or exercise (DOMS)
- Develop body awareness
- Promote circulation
- Improve relaxation within tense and tight muscles
- Aids stress relief

How to stretch correctly

There is no time limit to stretching, although do remember that less is best! The gentler you are with your stretching, the more you get out of the muscles.

When you find the first part of tension in your stretch, you should feel a really small amount, as if you are just about to stretch. It should be nice and simple and should isolate the muscle you are trying to focus on without involving any others. Allow the muscle adequate time to relax and elongate (there is no time limit).

If you are bouncing in stretches, feeling sharp pain in the muscle being stretched, feeling muscle spasm, shake or feel a burning sensation then you are probably stretching the muscle too hard and most likely, incorrectly. Remember, less is best!

There are different types of stretching which can improve flexibility, strength and are an important part in creating harmony within your body.

The Myo Stretch Routine enabled me to stretch all the muscles throughout my body over the 12-week plan. I repeated this every week to ensure an increase in muscle strength and resistance.

Static stretching

This means to perform a certain stretch without movement. This is when you find the first tension within the muscle and hold without moving from that position. Once it has released, you can either move onto the next stretch or gently repeat the action.

Developmental stretching

This works in the same way at the static stretch. You find the first point of tension and hold it until the muscle relaxes and elongates. Once you feel no stretch, go slightly further into the stretch until you feel tension for the second time. Repeat up to four times.

Proprioceptive Neuromusular Facilitation stretching or PNF

An advanced stretching and flexibility technique, that involves both the contraction and stretching of a muscle, this stretch is best performed with a professional or training partner although some can be tried at home. Always remember to listen to your body and take note on how to perform the PNF correctly.

To perform PNF Stretching:

1. Find the first bit of tension in the stretch and hold until the tension has elongated.

2. Contract the same muscle that was being stretched for 20-40% of your maximum effort (I always tend to push at 20%).

3. Hold the contraction of the muscle for 12 seconds.

4. Release the contraction and allowing the muscle to relax for a second.

5. Now find the second stretch by going further into the stretch until you find the tension again. (What you should have noticed was a greater range before feeling the stretch).

6. Again allow the stretch to relax and elongate before repeating the process.

7. You can repeat this process up to three times before coming out of the stretch.

Remember – do not use the PNF Stretch on muscles that are weak, elongated or overstretched.

1. Developmental stretch for calf (gastrocnemius) muscles

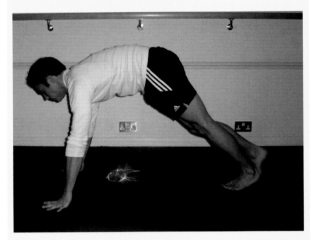

1. From a press up position, move your hand closer to your feet whilst raising your hips into the air.

2. With your feet together use one foot for support and the other foot should be flat on the floor with your legs extended straight, but not completely locked out.

3. Bend the leg that is for support.

4. Move your hands closer until you feel a small stretch in the calf of the foot that is flat to the ground.

5. Once the stretch has elongated, move your hands closer again to your feet, or you can push your heel into the floor. You should now be feeling a stretch in the middle part of your calf muscle.

6. Without dropping the position, allow your hands to go back to the starting position and repeat for the other leg. You will also be working your upper body whilst in this position.

7. Once you have completed the stretch on the other side, move your hands back to the start keeping in the same position. You are now ready to perform the soleus stretch.

2. Developmental stretch for soleus muscles

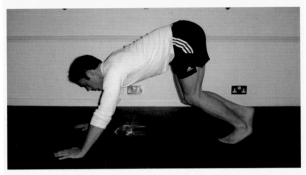

1. Stay in the position of the calf stretch – with your hands out in front of you and your hips in the air.

2. With your feet together, use one for support and the other almost flat on the floor, legs bent at the knee.

3. Move your hands closer until you feel a small stretch in the lower calf.

4. Once the stretch has elongated, move your hands closer to your feet, or you can push your heel into the floor. You should be feeling a stretch on the lower calf towards your Achilles' tendon.

5. Without dropping the position, allow your hands to go back to the starting position and repeat for the other leg. You will also be working your upper body whilst in this position.

6. Once you have completed the stretch on the other side, put both feet onto the floor and go back down into the press up position.

7. Sit up and sit back onto your heels. You are now ready to move onto the lower back stretch.

3. Static stretch for the lower back

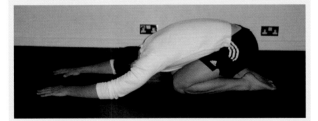

1. Whilst sitting on your heels, reach forwards from your hip with your hands out in front of you and let your head relax.

2. You should be nice and relaxed and you might be able to feel a stretch in your lower back and latissimus dorsi.

4. Developmental stretch for hip flexor stretch

Good stretch for a lordotic posture

1. Kneel on one foot.

2. If you need to, hold onto an object to help keep balance.

3. Lean slightly forwards so your weight is on the front foot.

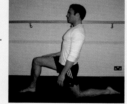

4. Push your hip out forwards.

5. To get more of a stretch, lean your torso slightly back in the opposite direction. You should feel a stretch in the front of your hip (iliacus, psoas major and rectus femoris).

6. From this position go straight into the PNF stretch on the same leg.

5. PNF stretch for hamstring muscles

Postural Stretch for flat back/sway back

1. Kneel on one knee with your other leg out in front so your foot is flat on the floor.

2. Keep your back straight whilst leaning forward to keep balance (you can either balance yourself with one or both arms down to the floor).

3. Sit back onto your knee.

4. Try to keep your leg out in front with a small bend in your knee.

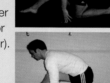

5. Tilt your buttocks up in the air to feel more of a stretch. As long as you have the stretch in your hamstrings you can now perform a PNF stretch if your muscle requires it.

6. Follow the same rule as how to perform a PNF stretch.

7. Whilst in the same position and now that the first stretch has released, you can now push your foot in the ground as if you were trying to curl your heel up to your bum. You should now feel the same muscle contract which was just being stretched (note; if you can't feel the contraction in your hamstring try moving until you do feel it).

8. Hold the contraction 20% of your maximal effort for 12 seconds.

9. Relax for one second and then move into the stretch for a second time.

10. Perform the PNF stretch 2 to 3 times. You should feel a stretch in the back of your thigh / hamstring (semimembranosus, semitendinosus and bicep femoris).

11. Sit back onto both of your heels.

12. Now change legs and repeat these last two stretches.

6. Static stretch for the lower back

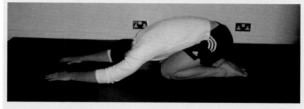

1. Whilst sitting on your heels reach forwards from your hip with your hands out in front of you and let your head relax.

2. You should be nice and relaxed, and you might be able to feel a stretch in your lower back and latissimus dorsi.

3. Sit back up onto your heels.

7. Developmental stretch for quad with your knees bent

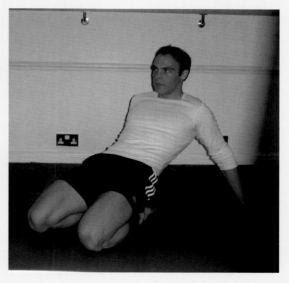

1. Whilst sitting on your heels, place your legs under your buttocks.

2. Lean back keeping your body weight on your arms.

3. You should then be able to feel a stretch in the middle part of your quads.

4. To feel more of a stretch or to develop the stretch move your hands further behind you or squeeze your glute muscles/ push out your hips. You should be able to feel a stretch within the middle part of your quads (rectus femoris, vastus medialis, vastus lateralis and vastus intermedius).

5. Roll over onto your front and lie face down.

8. PNF Stretch for quad lying face down

Posture stretch for lordotic postures

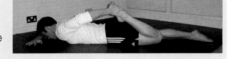

1. Lie face down.
2. Bring one foot up towards your buttock whilst holding onto it with the same side arm.
3. Pull the foot to your buttock to feel the stretch within the middle/upper part of the quad.
4. As long as you have the stretch in your quads you can now perform a PNF stretch if your muscle requires it. Follow the same rule as written in the 'How to perform a PNF stretch'.
5. Whilst in the same position and when the first stretch has released, you can now push your leg out as if you are trying to straighten it. You should now feel the same muscle contract. (If you can't, try to move slightly until you feel the muscle contract).
6. Hold the contraction 20% of your maximal effort for 12 seconds.
7. Relax for one second and then move into the stretch for a second time.
8. Perform the PNF stretch 2 to 3 times.
9. You should be able to feel a stretch within the middle to upper portion of the quads (rectus femoris, vastus medialis, vastus lateralis and the vastus intermedius).
10. Once you have stretched your quad swap your hands over so your opposite hand is on the leg being stretched.
11. From this position go straight into the static stretch for the quads on the same leg.

9. Static stretch for quad muscles lying down opposite hand to opposite leg

1. Lie face down.

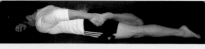

2. Bring one foot up towards your buttock whilst holding onto it with the opposite arm.
3. Pull the foot to your opposite buttock.
4. Keep your hips on the ground. You should be able to feel a stretch on the outer part of the quad).
5. Once you have finished stretching move onto your other leg and repeat.
6. Once you have finished your lying quad stretches you can relax for 1 or 2 minutes in this position.
7. Roll onto your back and sit up for your hamstring stretch.
8. Repeat these last two stretches on the other leg.

10. Developmental stretch for sitting hamstring muscles

Posture stretch for flat back or sway back

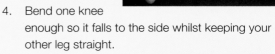

1. Place your arms on the ground besides you.
2. Place both legs out in front of you.
3. Sit with your back straight.
4. Bend one knee enough so it falls to the side whilst keeping your other leg straight.
5. Lean forwards from the hip until you find a stretch in your hamstrings. You should now be able to feel a stretch within your hamstring muscles (semimembranosus, semitendinosus and bicep femoris).
6. Once you have stretched one side move onto the other side.
7. When you have finished stretching your other leg, keep both legs out in front of you ready for the next stretch.

11. Developmental stretch for the wide leg adductor

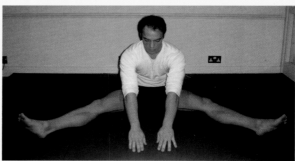

1. Sit with your legs straight out and wide in front of you (make sure it is as wide as you comfortably can so you don't feel a stretch on your hamstring muscles).
2. Sit with a straight back.
3. Lean forwards until you feel a stretch on your adductors. You should be able to feel inside of your thighs/ adductors (adductor longus, adductor brevis, adductor magnus and gracilis).
4. Bring both feet into your crutch and if possible with your feet together, to stretch adductors.

12. Developmental stretch for the sitting groin muscle

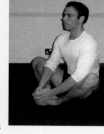

1. Sit with your back straight.
2. For support hold onto your feet.
3. Feet together if possible and allow your knees to drop out to the side.
4. You should feel a stretch on the inside of your thighs if not bring your feet in towards your groin.
5. You should be able to feel a stretch on the inside of your thighs / adductors (adductor longus, adductor brevis , adductor magnus and gracilis and pectineus).
6. Put both of your legs out in front of you and relax your body for one or two minutes.

13. Static stretch for sitting glute muscle extensions

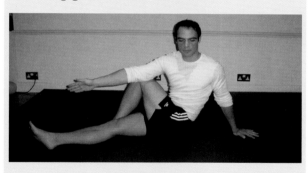

1. Sit with one leg out straight and cross the other leg over your knee.
2. Turn your shoulders around so your torso is facing away from your body.
3. Place one arm onto your raised knee to help you rotate around even further and your other arm out behind you to support yourself. You should be able to feel a stretch in your glute muscles (gluteus maximus, gluteus medius and gluteus minimus) as well as tensor fasciae latae and piriformis.
4. Good stretch if you feel pain in your lower back.
5. Swap your legs over to stretch your other side.
6. Keep your leg crossed but relaxed. Roll back onto your back to stretch your deeper glute muscles.
7. Change your legs over and repeat the same stretch.

14. Developmental stretch for glute muscles

Postural Stretch when suffering from sciatica (caused by your piriformis being too tight)

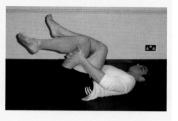

1. Lie on your back on the floor face up.
2. Cross one leg over the other leg.
3. Start to bring your foot down towards your buttock.
4. Grasp onto the thigh (hamstrings) just under the knee.
5. Pull the leg up and towards your chest. You should be able to feel a stretch in your glute muscles (piriformis, deep glute muscles and gluteus maximus).
6. Stretch the other side then relax with your feet on the ground and your knees in the air.
7. Bring both knees into your chest to stretch your lower back.
8. Change your legs over and repeat the stretch on the other side.

15. Developmental stretch for the lower back whilst lying down

Postural stretch if you have a Lordotic posture

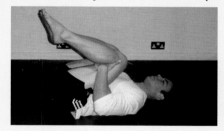

1. Lie on your back, face up.
2. Hold onto the back of both of your thighs, just underneath the knees.
3. Pull your knees towards your chest, allowing your buttocks to rise off the ground. You should be able to feel a stretch in your lower back and gluteus maximus.
4. Once the stretch has released, drop your feet on the floor with knees bent and relaxed.
5. Drop legs flat to the floor for the next stretch.

16. Static stretch for the whole body

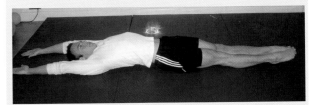

1. Lie on your back and extend your legs out straight in front of you and your arms out straight overhead.

2. Now lengthen your body as much as possible by pointing your toes and pushing your arms overhead. You should be able to feel a stretch in different places of the body (including your abs, serratus anterior, lattisimus dorsi, etc).

3. Once the stretch has relaxed, bring your arms out to your side for the next stretch.

17. Static stretch for lying roll over

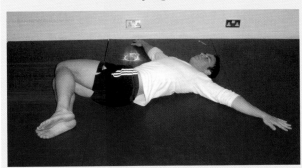

1. Lie on your back.

2. Keep your arms out to your side and bring your knees up with your feet on the floor.

3. Allow your knees to drop to one side and try to relax your back and hips to get the best stretch. You should be able to feel a stretch in your lower back muscles and glute muscles.

4. Bring your knee back up to the centre and drop to the other side.

5. Stay on your back in a relaxed position and relax for two to three minutes.

6. Roll onto your front for the abdominal stretch.

18. Static stretch for the abdominal muscles
Postural Stretch for flat back

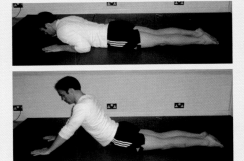

1. Lie face down onto the floor.

2. Keeping your hands in front of you, about shoulder width apart.

3. Keep your hips, legs and feet flat on the ground.

4. Raise your torso off the ground until your arms are almost straight or you feel a stretch in your abdominals.

5. Hold this stretch for no longer than 10 seconds.

19. Static stretch for the oblique muscles

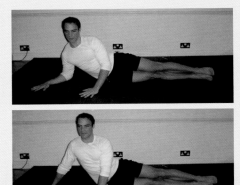

1. Lie on your side keeping your body straight.

2. Make sure the leg you're resting is touching the whole of the floor.

3. With your forearm resting on the floor and your other arm in front of you for support, extend your resting arm out straight so your body weight is resting on your hand instead.

4. You should now feel a stretch on your side. You should be able to feel a stretch in your oblique muscles.

5. Roll onto your front and then onto the other side to stretch your other obliques.

6. Once you have stretched your other side roll back onto your front for the cat stretch.

20. Static cat stretch

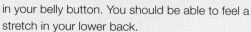

1. Kneel on all fours.

2. Let your head fall forwards and relax.

3. Arch your back and draw in your belly button. You should be able to feel a stretch in your lower back.

4. Relax from your stretch and then sit back onto heels for another lower back stretch

21. Static stretch for the lower back

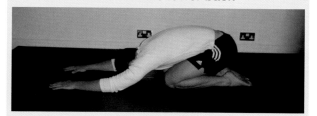

1. Whilst sitting on your heels reach forwards from your hip with your hands out in front of you and let your head relax. You should be nice and relaxed and you might be able to feel a stretch in your lower back and latissimus dorsi.

2. Stay in this position, you're ready to get onto the next stretch.

22. Development lat stretch on the floor

1. Sitting on your heels reach forwards with your hands.

2. Place one arm across your body with it resting onto the floor.

3. Use your fingers to walk your arm diagonally away from your body to feel a stretch in your latissimus dorsi.

4. Keep walking your fingers out to get a developmental stretch.

5. Bring your arm back to the centre and then swap over to the other side.

23. Static stretch for the bicep muscles

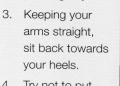

1. Kneel on all fours.

2. Turn your arms so the inside of your forearms are facing away from you and your fingers are pointing at you.

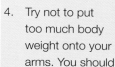

3. Keeping your arms straight, sit back towards your heels.

4. Try not to put too much body weight onto your arms. You should feel a stretch on the front of the top of your arms (bicep and you also might feel a stretch on your wrist flexors).

5. Sit back up onto your heels and relax for two to three minutes.

24. Static stretch for the triceps muscles

1. Sit on your heels.

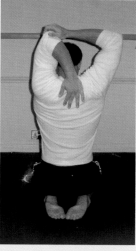

2. Place one hand up and behind your head with your elbow pointing upwards.

3. With your other hand (depending on your flexibility) either pull the elbow down from the top or you can push the elbow from the front. You should be able to feel a stretch on the back of your upper arm (triceps).

4. Now stand up for the final stretches – you can move around to get the blood flowing around your muscles.

5. Follow the next stretches one after the other whilst standing.

25. Static stretch for wrist flexor muscles

1. With one hand, hold onto the fingers of your other hand and straighten your arm so your forearm is facing upwards.

2. Pull your fingers/hand towards your body. You should be able to feel a stretch on the inside of your forearm.

3. Repeat this stretch on your other hand.

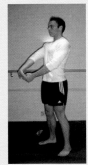

26. Static stretch for the wrist extensor muscles

1. With one hand, hold onto the opposite fingers/hand and straighten your arm so your forearm is facing down.

2. Pull your fingers/hand towards your body. You should be able to feel a stretch on the back of your forearm.

3. Repeat this stretch on your other hand.

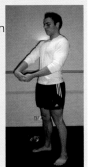

27. Static stretch for the anterior deltoid muscles

1. Place your hands into the base of your back.

2. Drop your shoulders forwards and raise up your chest, as if you're taking in a deep breathe. You should be able to feel a stretch at the front of your shoulders (anterior deltoid).

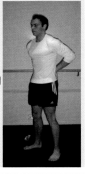

28. Static stretch for the deltoid muscles

1. Place one arm across the front of your body.

2. You can either keep that arm straight or you can bend it to a 90 degree angle.

3. Pull your arm in and towards the opposite arm until you feel a stretch. You should be able to feel a stretch in your shoulder and slightly in the upper back (rear deltoid, rhomboids, and trapezius).

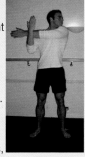

29. Static stretch for the chest with hands behind the back

1. Place your hands into the base of your spine.

2. Bring your elbows as close together as possible and push your chest out. You should be able to feel a stretch in your chest (pectoral major, pectoral minor, anterior deltoid).

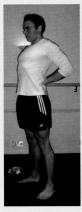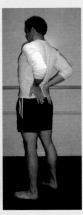

30. Static stretch for the chest on a wall
Postural stretch for Kyphotic posture.

1. Stand beside a wall, with your feet shoulder width apart.

2. Bend your arm to a 90 degree angle at the elbow and rest your forearm onto the wall or door frame.

3. Place the same side leg forwards.

4. Turn your body and shoulders away from the bent arm until you feel a stretch in your chest (pectoral major, pectoral minor, anterior deltoid).

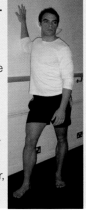

31. Static stretch for the lat muscle

1. Place your feet shoulder-width apart and extend one arm across your body in front of you.

2. Reach across as far as possible with your hands whilst leaning slightly forwards.

3. The key is to try and arch the side of your back.

4. You can vary this by holding onto an object or doorway (This will give you a deeper stretch into the lat muscle). You should be able to feel a stretch in the side of your back (latissimus dorsi).

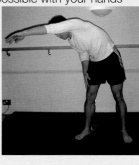

32. Static stretch for the rhomboid muscles

1. Place your hands together in front of you about shoulder height.

2. Reach forwards as far as comfortable with your hands, trying to round the middle/upper part of your back. You should be able to feel a stretch in the middle of your upper back between your shoulder blades (rhomboids).

3. It's just like hugging a tree!

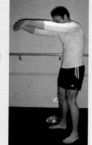

33. Static stretch for the trapezius muscles

This can sometimes help Kyphotic postures if you are feeling pain in the neck

1. Whilst looking straight ahead, allow your head (ear) to drop towards the shoulder on the same side.

2. Keep your hands behind your back to get the best stretch. You should be able to feel a stretch on

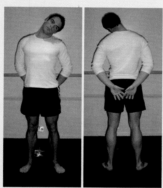

the top of your shoulders into your neck (trapezius, levator scapulae).

Ending the Myo Stretch routine

To finish the routine, stand on your tip toes and extend your arms overhead nice and straight. You should be able to feel a stretch throughout your body and then release. Take a little walk around to get the blood moving throughout your whole body, including moving your arms.

You have now completed the Myo Stretch routine and should feel relaxed, with no tension in your body.

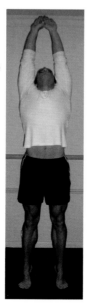

Your Next Steps

This General Health Guide is just one part of the Train to Become series. In order to get the maximum results from your 12-week plan, use it in conjunction with the Train to Become Fitness and Nutrition books to do the Train to Become Challenge. These books clearly show that with commitment and determination, you too can achieve a healthier and happier you!

If you need a little extra support or would like some additional advice, please visit my website at **www.traintobecome.com** and feel free to contact me by email at **contact@traintobecome.com**.

Train to Become Challenge

The Train to Become Challenge has been designed for you to follow all three books for the 12 weeks. During this time you will have gained all the knowledge necessary to get your body in to its best shape ever!

Do not just take my word for it. You can see the results for yourself in the pictures in all the books in the series.

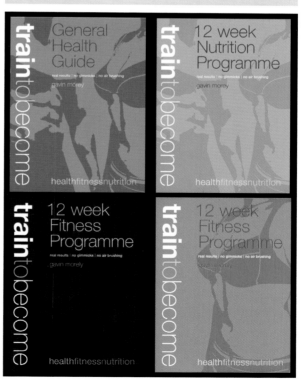

Index